# BIPOLAR BASICS

## Unpacking the Nuances and Understanding Solutions

Tracey Marks, MD

Bipolar Basics: Unpacking the Nuances and Understanding Solutions
Copyright © 2021 by Tracey Marks, MD
All rights reserved.

Printed in the United States of America

First Edition 2021
Book design by Nebojsa Dolovacki

ISBN 978-1-7366509-0-5 (paperback)
ISBN 978-1-7366509-1-2 (ebook)
Library of Congress Control Number: 2021903261

Trademarks, Legal Notice and Disclaimer

Dr. Tracey Marks
6525 The Corners Pkwy, Ste 212
Peachtree Corners, GA 30092

www.MarksPsychiatry.com

# BIPOLAR BASICS—UNPACKING THE NUANCES AND UNDERSTANDING SOLUTIONS

## BIPOLAR DISORDER'S NUANCES

## TREATMENT OPTIONS

## COMPARISON OF SIMILAR CONDITIONS

# Introduction

Ten years ago, I set out to demystify mental health by using YouTube to present educational videos about mental health topics. My goal was to present information in a way that could be easily understood. It took me a while to get off the ground but, by 2018, I finally started producing content consistently. Based on feedback from viewers, the information benefited many people in practical ways.

It's been fulfilling, to say the least, to generate a library of information that advances the understanding of mental disorders, their treatments, and their relationship to behavior. I'm excited about the opportunity to continue down this path.

Writing this handbook was inspired by my viewers. Many have commented that they take notes on the videos to reference later, and many of the video topics were explicitly developed in direct response to their questions.

To that end, I've chosen the top 25 videos from 2018 to 2021 related to bipolar disorder and organized them for this handbook to use as a written resource. I hope you find it valuable.

Still, it's important to note that this is just an informational resource. It's not meant to be a substitute for seeing a doctor or mental health specialist. In the treatment section, I discuss medication options and non-medication strategies. This is still for educational purposes and not meant to be medical advice or to establish a doctor-patient relationship.

# THE NUANCES OF BIPOLAR DISORDER

## CHAPTER 1

# What is Bipolar Disorder and What Do Mania and Hypomania Really Look Like?

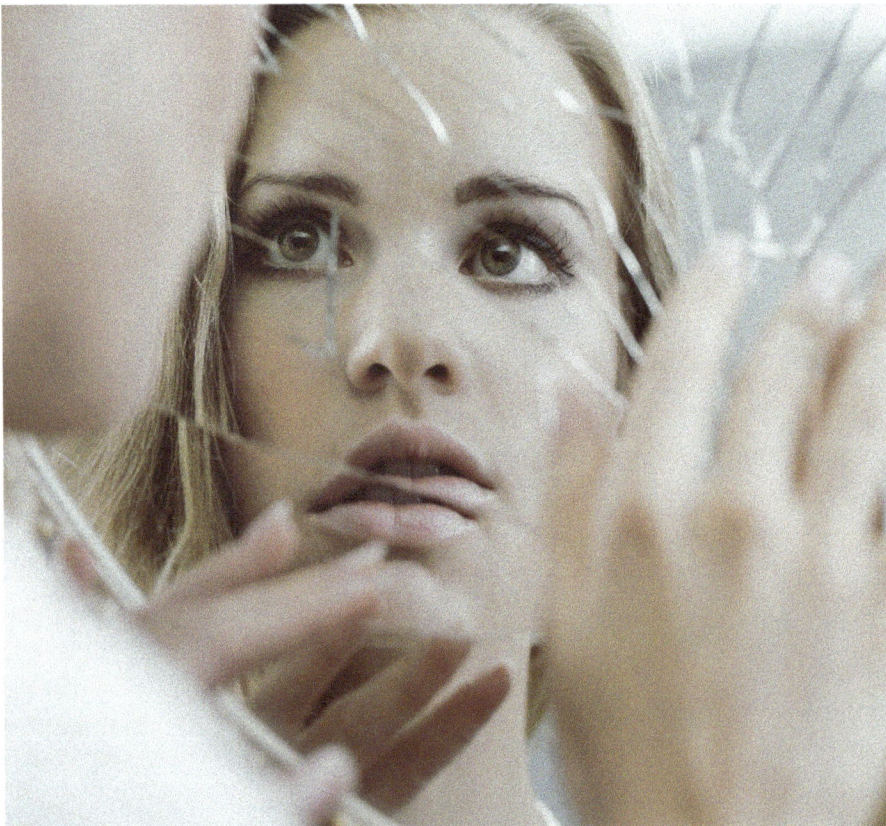

Bipolar disorder is a mood disorder that can present with episodes of depression or mania. Both bipolar disorder and major depressive disorder have bouts of depression.

**B**ut hypomania and mania are really the defining characteristics of bipolar disorder and set it apart from depression (sometimes referred to as unipolar depression).

If you're wondering if you have bipolar disorder, the first question you and your doctor or therapist have to answer is whether you've actually had a manic episode.

Here's an example of how that question can look practically. John goes to see his doctor and says he hasn't felt well for years. His close friend told him he should really look into whether he has a bipolar disorder because he's been depressed for years and it keeps coming back.

A common misconception is that if you have depression that keeps coming back, it must be bipolar disorder.

The first question to ask is: **what does your mania or hypomania look like? If you've never been**

**manic or hypomanic, it's not bipolar disorder, at least not currently.**

Here's how a manic episode is defined using the *Diagnostic and Statistical Manual of Mental Disorders*, 5th edition:

*A distinct period of abnormally and persistently elevated, expansive, or irritable mood along with abnormally and persistently increased activity or energy, lasting at least one week and present most of the day, nearly every day (or any duration if you need to go to the hospital).*

Before we go any further, let's break this down.

The key terms are "abnormally" and "persistently." You have mood changes and energy and activity changes that are abnormal. Sometimes experiencing happiness feels abnormal when you've not been happy in a while. But mania is more than feeling happy. This criterion refers to happiness or irritability that's over-the-top to the extent

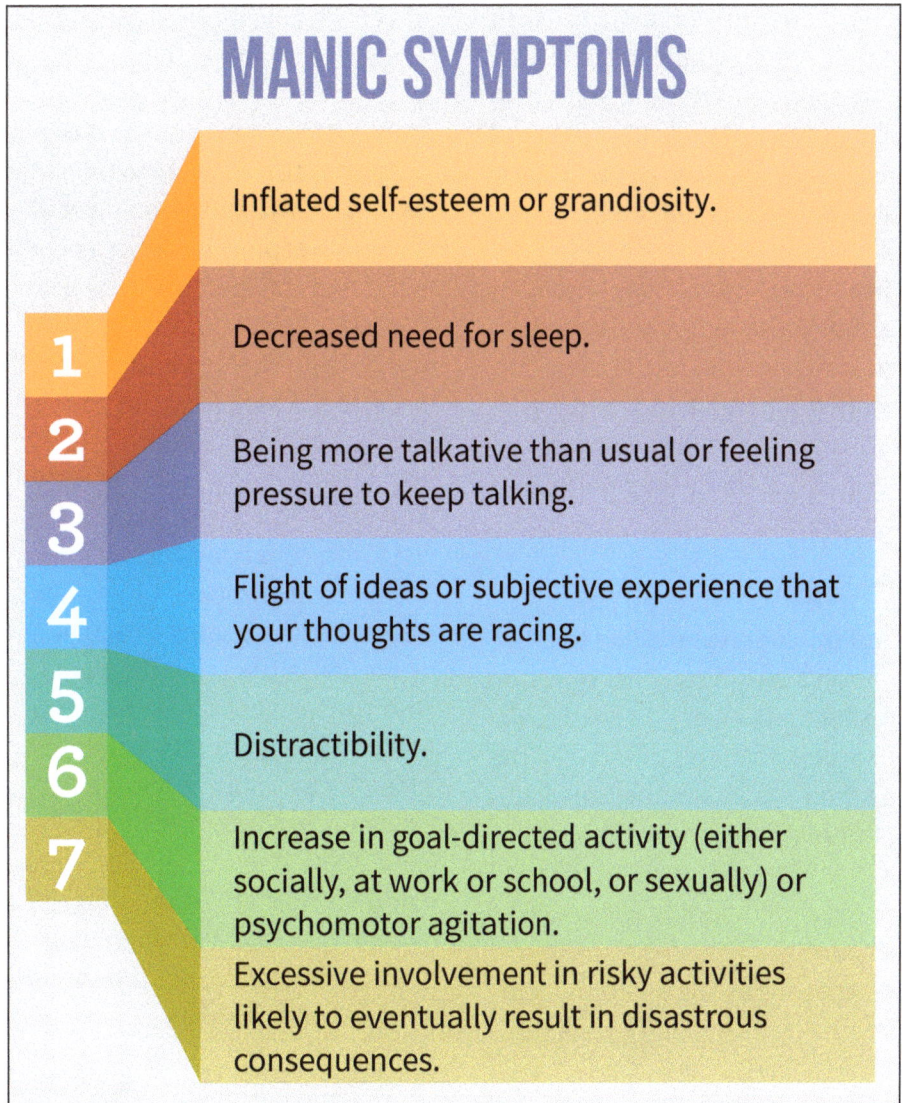

# MANIC SYMPTOMS

1. Inflated self-esteem or grandiosity.

2. Decreased need for sleep.

3. Being more talkative than usual or feeling pressure to keep talking.

4. Flight of ideas or subjective experience that your thoughts are racing.

5. Distractibility.

6. Increase in goal-directed activity (either socially, at work or school, or sexually) or psychomotor agitation.

7. Excessive involvement in risky activities likely to eventually result in disastrous consequences.

> HYPOMANIA IS A CONSTELLATION OF SYMPTOMS LASTING A MINIMUM OF FOUR DAYS, AS DEFINED BY THE *DSM*.

that people notice and think it's abnormal. Because "abnormal" is a relative term, another way to think of it is whether your emotions or behavior stands out to others.

This might look like planning to run for president, even though you're woefully unqualified for the job, or experiencing an on-top-of-the-world feeling where you believe you can bring an end to world hunger with an idea you just developed. You may stay up all or most of the night working on projects and do this multiple nights in a row.

What does the increased energy or activity look like? This is more than feeling motivated to go to the gym four days in a row and then "crashing" and not returning. That four days you went to the gym isn't evidence of manic behavior.

Instead, it might look like spending 4–5 hours each day at the gym, and you're fifty years old. If you're doing that at twenty, it may not be abnormal. It could also look like excessive organizing and cleaning. If you have family visiting and you need to spend all week cleaning your house, it doesn't mean you're manic. With mania, you would engage in an excessive or abnormal amount of cleaning that generally has some negative impact (e.g., you're not sleeping as a result, etc.).

The second part of this criterion is that these mood and energy changes need to last at least one week for mania and four days for hypomania. Both can last longer, but that's the minimum timeframe.

Suppose you wake up one day and think that you'd like to be a nation's president. Then you start researching what you need to do to accomplish this objective.  The next day you abandon the plan after realizing it just won't work. In this instance, you didn't have one day of mania or hypomania. Hypomania is a constellation of symptoms lasting a minimum of four days, as defined by the *DSM*.

## THE NEXT PART OF THE CRITERIA

During this period of mood change and increased energy or activity, you must have at least three of the following seven symptoms. If your abnormal mood is irritable, then you need four of the seven symptoms. These are things constituting a noticeable change from your usual behavior.

**1   Inflated self-esteem or grandiosity.** This goes back to the example of knowing you're going to be president, despite having no political support or a reasonable chance of getting anywhere close to achieving this objective.

**2   Decreased need for sleep.** This could mean going a few days without sleeping at all or sleeping 2 to 3 hours each night and still feeling rested the next day. This is different from trying to go to sleep and having trouble sleeping because you're worried about a deadline you need to meet. Nor is it staying up late while you review your to-do list for the next day. Instead, it means losing track of time while you're busy engaging in activities without realizing that it's 4 am, and you never got in bed to go to sleep. If you go to bed, you only sleep for a couple of hours then wake up, ready for the next day.

For this criterion, the operative phrase is a departure from your usual behavior. If you're someone who works or studies a lot of hours and routinely sleeps 3 to 4 hours every night, then your poor sleep isn't a sign of mania. It's just your usual sleep pattern.

**3   Being more talkative than usual or feeling pressure to keep talking.** Some people are generally more talkative. In fact, some people with ADHD can be very conversational or have some degree of uninterruptible speech (called pressured). We'll look at the comparison between ADHD and bipolar disorder in Chapter 24.

The kind of pressured speech you see with mania tends to be more noticeable to others, whereas, from your vantage point, it doesn't appear to be a problem at all. In your mind, you've got a lot to say, and the ideas keep flowing. The person listening experiences this conversation as

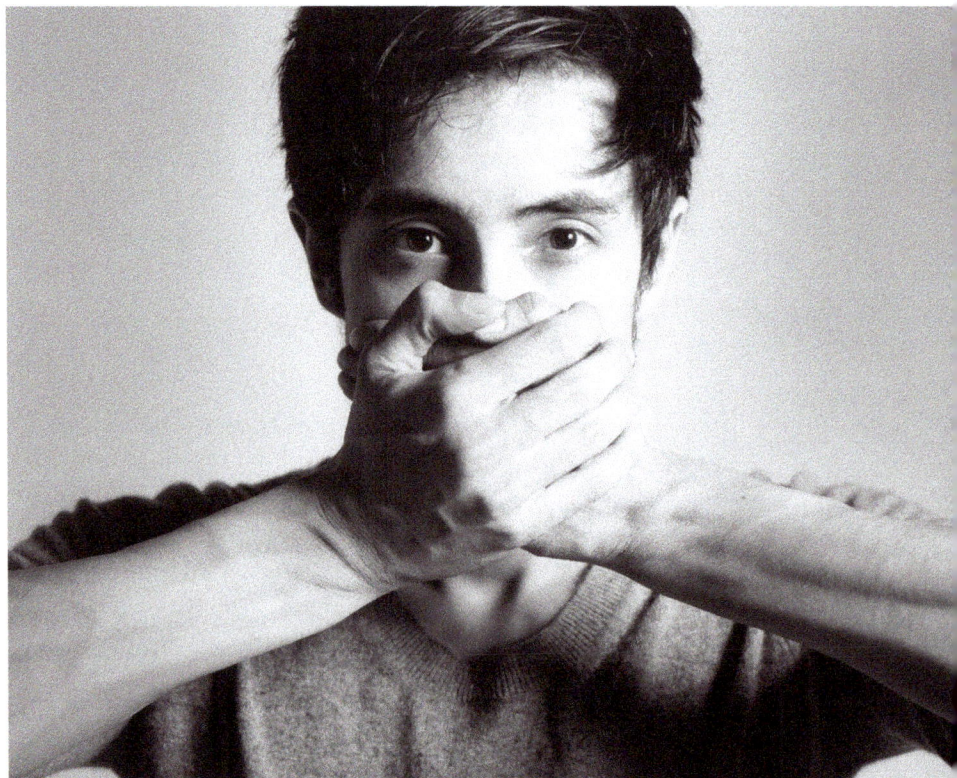

> WITH HYPOMANIA, YOU MAY STILL BE ABLE TO GO TO WORK OR SCHOOL. THE SYMPTOMS ARE STILL NOTICEABLE TO OTHERS, BUT THEY'RE NOT AS SEVERE.

an unwelcome assault of words. They feel trapped behind a wall of talking.

That experience is different from talking to a person who's just talkative. The hyperverbal person is usually interruptible. But with mania or hypomania, it's hard to jump in and interrupt because there's no natural break in the conversation.

**4** **Flight of ideas or subjective experience that your thoughts are racing.** As your mania ramps up, it can get to where your racing thoughts outpace your ability to keep up with them. Internally you experience it as your mind moving so fast that you can barely think clearly.  This is what we refer to as a flight of ideas. Your thoughts are moving a mile a minute. The fast pace doesn't feel productive, though, because your thoughts are often disjointed.

**5** **Distractibility.** Here, unimportant or irrelevant external things easily draw your attention.

**6** **Increase in goal-directed activity (either socially, at work or school, or sexually) or psychomotor agitation.** These actions are purposeless and non-goal-directed.

Psychomotor agitation can look like pacing or lots of fidgeting when you're sitting. Or it can look like getting up to do things but not really doing anything. You may look busy, going in and out of rooms or in and out of the house while you accomplish nothing. If a person asks you what you're doing, you may not be able to give a meaningful answer because you're not actually sure what you were intending to do. But you can't feel settled.  You feel anxious. You don't feel nervous. But you feel as if you have to move and do things.

**7** **Excessive involvement in risky activities likely to eventually result in disastrous consequences.** Examples of this would be buying sprees, engaging in sexual indiscretions, or undertaking foolish business investments.

Hypersexuality is addressed in Chapter 9.

So, here, we have an abnormal mood and abnormal energy level along with three or four things from the list above.

With all these things happening simultaneously, serious problems surface in your social life or occupational or school functioning. You may even require

hospitalization to keep you from harming yourself or others.

You may also have psychotic features in the form of hallucinations or delusions. A common kind of delusion is called "ideas of reference" or "delusions of reference." Here, a person will believe that unrelated things have personal significance. For example, you may believe the radio or television is speaking to you.  This is different than hearing the television say something it didn't say—that is an auditory hallucination.

With ideas of reference, you hear what's being said and assign a different meaning to it that lines up with a delusion you already have. Here's an example. You believe your coworkers are trying to get you fired.  Whenever you hear someone say "projections," it's a confirmation signal in your mind that the person is in a ring of people who are conspiring to get you fired. You see the use of this word as a hidden message that your days are numbered. Even though you work for a marketing company where this word is frequently used, you are convinced that "projections" is a secret code word. This is one example of ideas of reference and how delusions can manifest in mania.

## HYPOMANIA VS. MANIA

Hypomania involves having all of the same criteria, except the symptoms only need to last for 4 days, and they don't cause the same problems with your functioning. With hypomania, you may still be able to go to work or school. The symptoms are still noticeable to others, but they're not as severe.

In fact, some people enjoy hypomania because it's a relief from their depression. While hypomanic, you may still look amped up to others, but it may not be causing you a problem. Also, usually with hypomania, you don't need hospitalization, and you're not doing things like,

say, showing up to work naked. With hypomania, you don't depart from reality and become psychotic. Psychosis is a severity indicator. If you have psychosis, it's mania.

Real mania or hypomania is usually apparent. People can feel the energy in the room. Sometimes you may be talking loudly, and the people in earshot think you're angry or yelling. But you're not angry. You're just talking. But because there's so much power behind your voice

because of your energy and enthusiasm, it comes off to others as if you're yelling or agitated.

### When is it called bipolar 1 instead of bipolar 2?

If you have a manic episode, your diagnosis is bipolar disorder, type 1. If you have a hypomanic episode, your diagnosis is bipolar disorder, type 2, and you'll have recurring episodes of hypomania and depression.

When you have a full manic episode, your diagnosis remains bipolar 1 even if your future episodes are hypomania. However, if you have multiple episodes of hypomania and depression and then have a more severe manic episode with psychosis, your bipolar 2 diagnosis will change to bipolar 1. So, you can "upgrade" from 2 to 1 but can't downgrade from 1 to 2.

Still, when you're looking at the big picture, it doesn't matter whether your diagnosis is bipolar 1 or 2, because the treatment is mostly the same. What's different is the course of the illness and how much time you will spend in a depressed state. People with bipolar 1 can have recurring manic episodes back to back and few depressive episodes, whereas people with bipolar 2 can have more prolonged and more frequent depressive episodes. This will be addressed in Chapter 4.

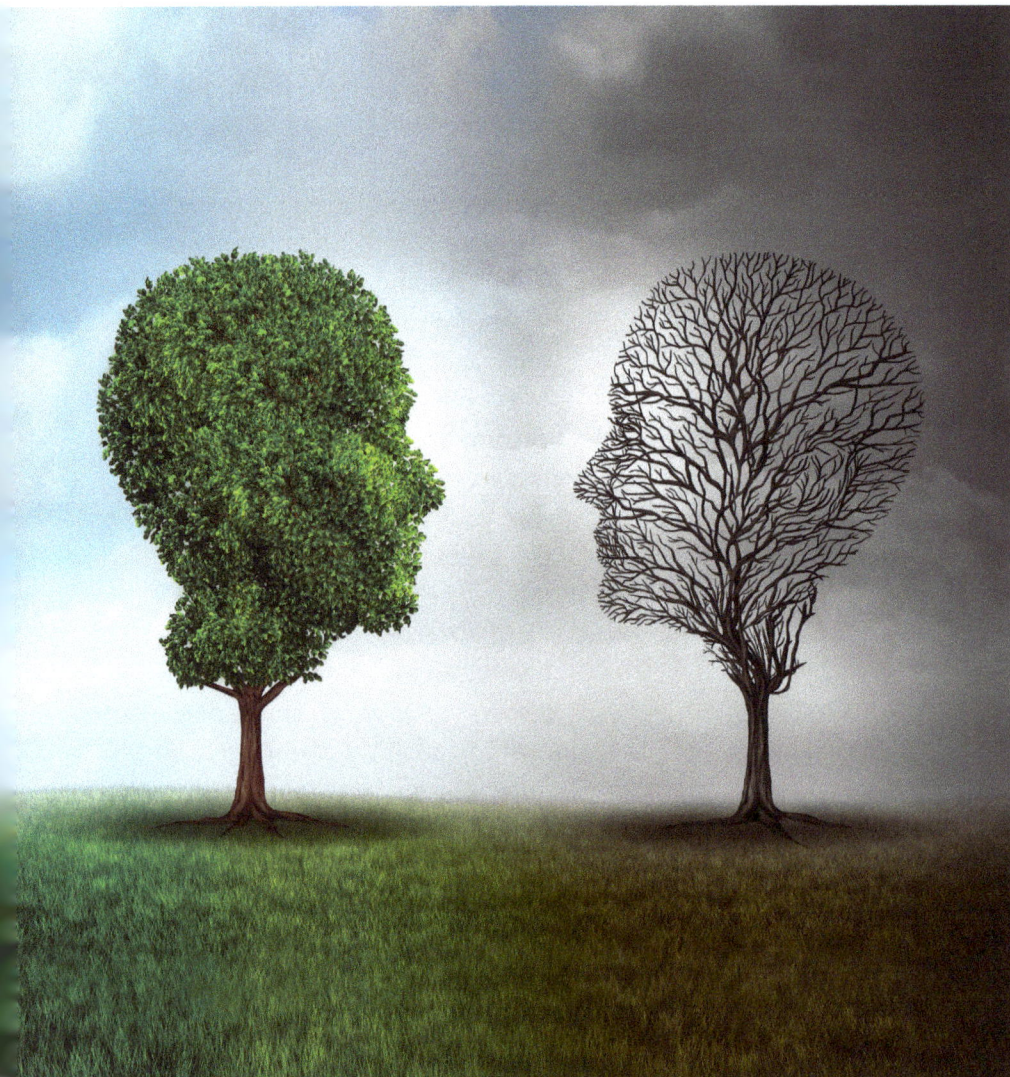

## CHAPTER 2

# How To Tell If You're Depressed

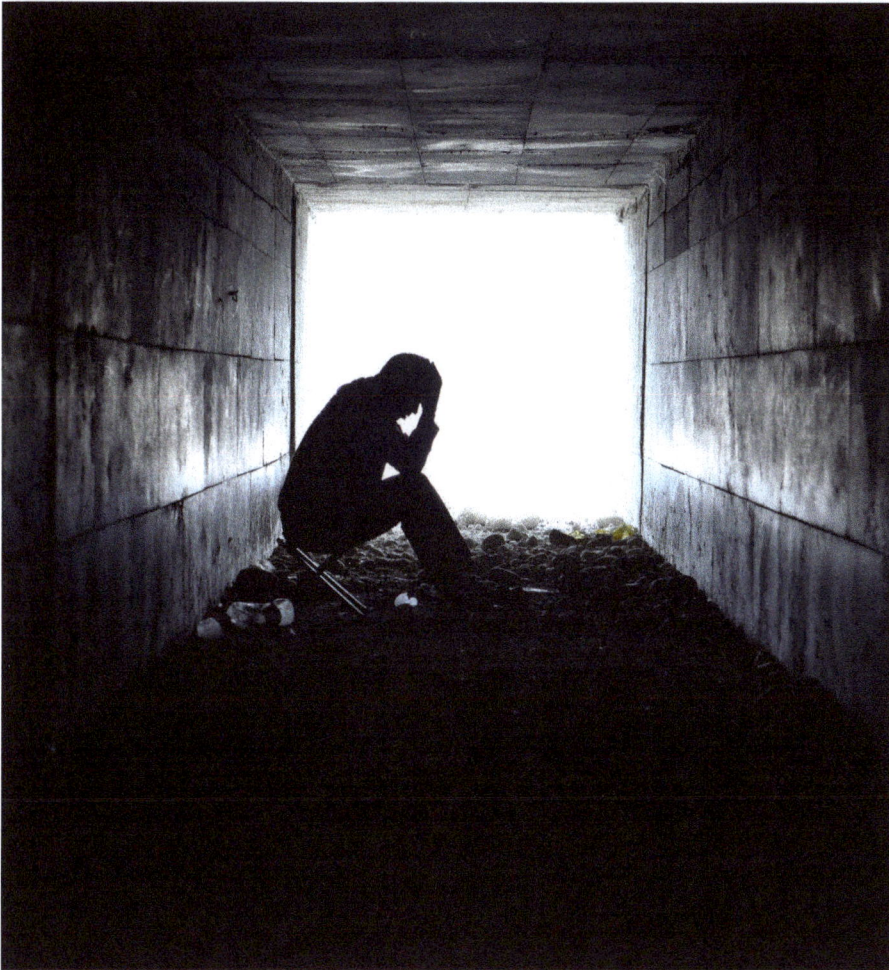

Sometimes it can be hard to tell if you have clinical depression or a temporary sadness or absence of mania. Some people, when things have slowed down from mania, question whether the lack of excitement is a depressed state.

Here is how depression is defined by the *Diagnostic and Statistical Manual of Mental Disorders*, 5th edition (*DSM*). The *DSM* is the textbook that clinicians use to diagnose mental disorders. There is no blood test or brain scan to prove you have depression, but there are clusters of symptoms that have been studied and shown to be present in people with depression.

For depression, you must have five of the following symptoms for at least two weeks. All of these

We've talked a lot about mania and hypomania because those states establish the difference between major depressive disorder (also referred to as unipolar depression) and bipolar disorder. But how do you know if you're depressed?

WITH DEPRESSION, YOU CAN QUICKLY BECOME OVERWHELMED BY HAVING TO THINK ABOUT OPTIONS.

symptoms must be present most of the day and nearly every day. So, they're not fleeting feelings.

**1 Depressed mood**
You may feel sad, hopeless, or even empty. You can also feel angry and irritable. It may be more common for children or adolescents to be irritable beyond what would be expected from childhood upset or teenage moodiness.

**2 Lack of enjoyment**
We call this anhedonia. You can't seem to find pleasure in things you used to enjoy.

**3 Weight loss or gain of 5% or a decrease or increase in appetite**

**4 Insomnia or hypersomnia**
With insomnia, you have trouble falling or staying asleep and usually sleep less than 5 hours in total.

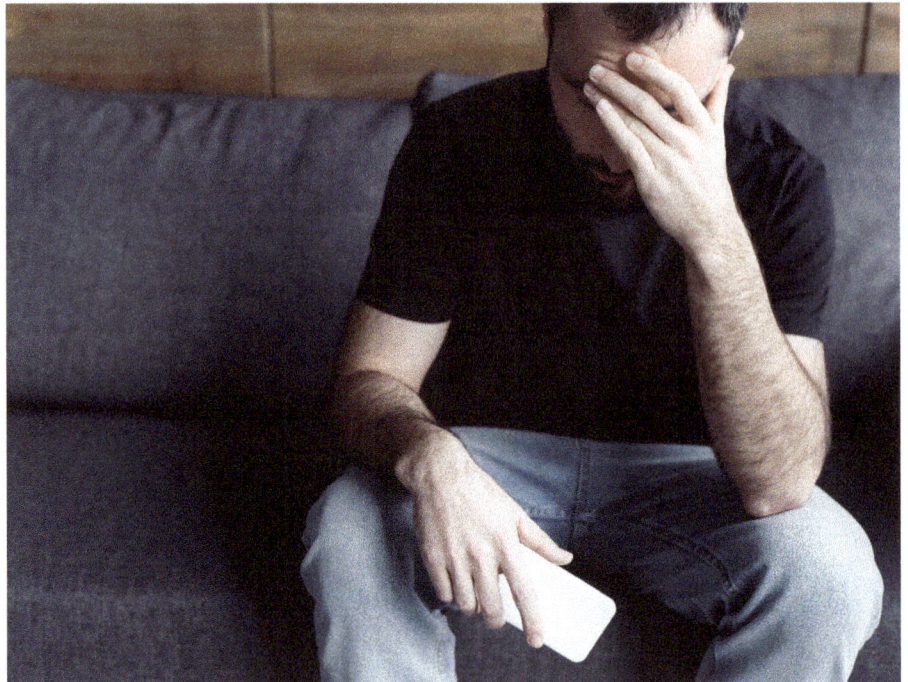

Hypersomnia involves sleeping more than 10 hours. This could be continuous or a total of your nightly sleep and naps.

**5 Being slowed or restless**
Some have noted they can tell when their depression is coming because their limbs feel heavy.

**6 Feeling tired or having low energy every day**

**7 Feeling worthless or excessively guilty**
With this symptom, you may feel responsible for all the wrong you see around you. You may even experience thought loops where you keep running over in your mind where things went wrong or how you should have kept something from happening. Some people can get so preoccupied with this train of thought that they become overly critical of themselves.

**8 Having trouble thinking, concentrating, or making decisions**
Depression is a massive disruptor to your ability to concentrate and focus. If you can't focus or pay attention, you'll have trouble remembering things.

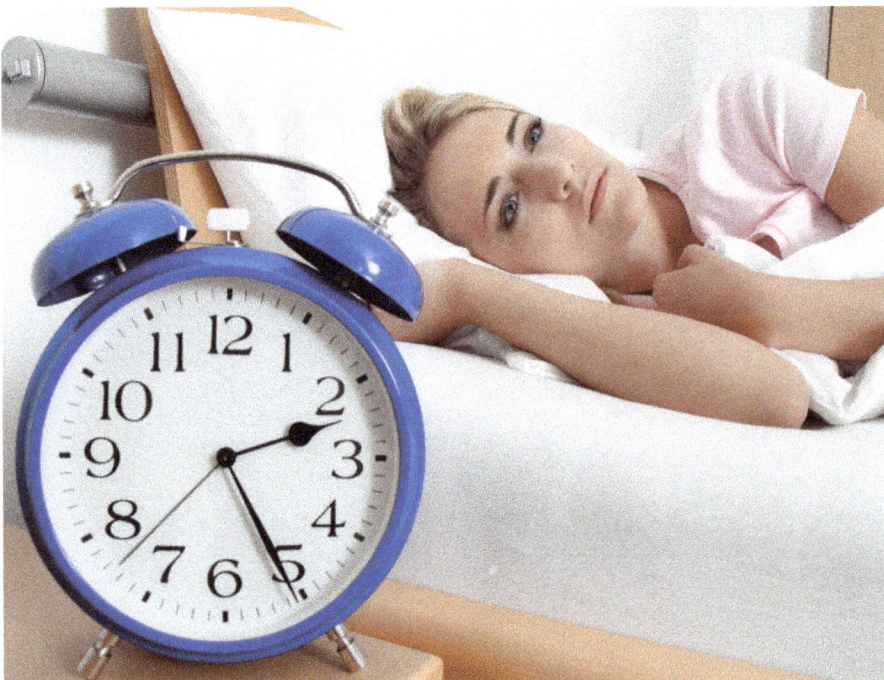

## SYMPTOMS OF DEPRESSION

**1** Depressed mood

**2** Lack of enjoyment

**3** Weight loss or gain of 5% or a decrease or increase in appetite

**4** Insomnia or hypersomnia

**5** Being slowed or restless

**6** Feeling tired or having low energy every day

**7** Feeling worthless or excessively guilty

**8** Having trouble thinking, concentrating, or making decisions

**9** Thinking about death, or thinking about dying by suicide.

> **AN EPISODE OF DEPRESSION REQUIRES FIVE OF THOSE SYMPTOMS OCCURRING AT THE SAME TIME.**

Therefore, depression can lead to memory problems.

Indecision has been seen as one of the core symptoms that most people have during depression. It's thought to be partly related to poor focus and problem-solving and partly related to not seeing the reward for your effort. With depression, you can quickly become overwhelmed by having to think about options. That can translate to not being able to get started with a plan. The effort that it takes to analyze the situation and forecast how the decision affects you is just too much to work through.

**9 Thinking about death, or thinking about dying by suicide**

Depression can distort your perception of your future. Things can look really bleak and may even get to the point where you just want to end the pain.

There's a difference between passive suicidality and active suicidality. Here's an example. Suppose you were crossing the street and had this thought: "If a car hit me right now, I'd be okay with that." That's passive suicidality. You have no plan or intention of ending your life, but the prospect of something ending your life is attractive.

People are actively suicidal when they start formulating a plan in their head, even though at the moment they're holding back from acting on it. Active suicidality is an emergency and should be treated in a hospital or crisis center setting until you're stable.

An episode of depression requires at least five of those symptoms occurring at the same time. With severe depression, you may develop psychotic symptoms such as delusions or hallucinations. Some research suggests that developing psychosis during the depressed phase increases the chance that you'll later develop bipolar disorder.

## CHAPTER 3

# Five Signs That You Likely Have Bipolar Disorder, Not Major Depression

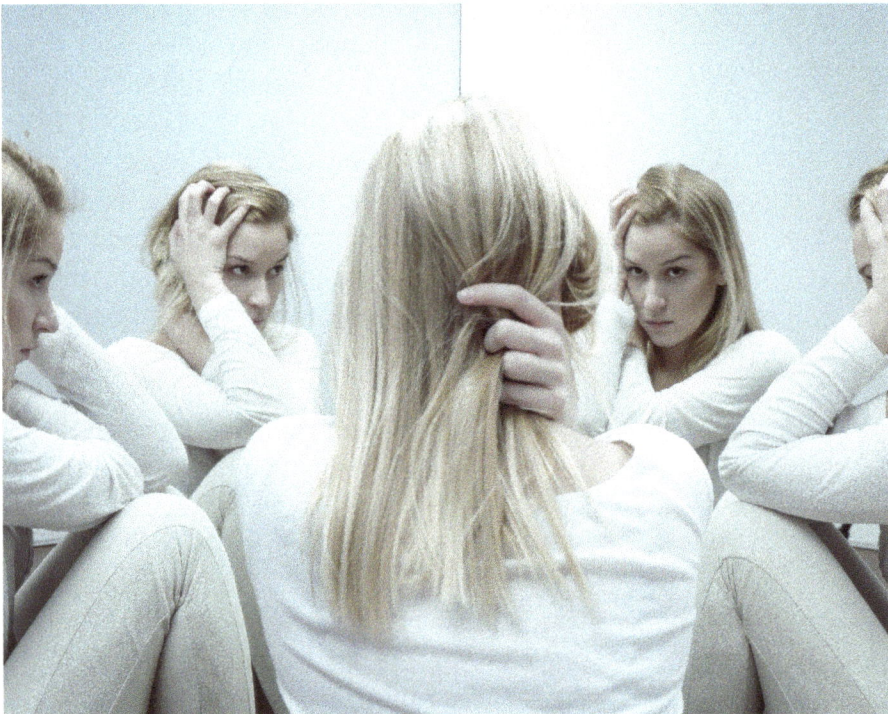

**B**ut there may be some signs that your depression is really bipolar disorder, even though you haven't yet been diagnosed with it. This is significant because the treatment for bipolar disorder is different from the treatment for unipolar depression.

Here are five signs that you may really be on the bipolar spectrum. This information is based on criteria outlined in the *DSM* and the Bipolarity Index by Dr. Gary Sachs.

Bipolar disorder can often start with a depressive episode. If this is the case, you may have a diagnosis of major depression for years until you have your first manic or hypomanic episode. Then your diagnosis will change to bipolar or 1 or 2.

{ BIPOLAR DISORDER IS CYCLICAL AND TENDS TO RETURN ON A SOMEWHAT REGULAR OR FREQUENT BASIS. }

## FIVE SIGNS THAT YOU'RE ON THE BIPOLAR SPECTRUM

**1** Your first depressive episode occurs before the age of 20

**2** Antidepressants sometimes don't work and can make things worse

**3** You have a family member with bipolar disorder

**4** You have three or more depressive episodes over five years

**5** You take a mood stabilizer and have a full recovery within one month

antidepressant in the past, but they may stop working as you get closer to having your first manic or mixed episode.

**3 You have a family member with bipolar disorder**

This is more significant when the family member is a first-degree relative, like a parent or sibling, instead of a more distant relative, such as a cousin.

**4 You have three or more depressive episodes over five years**

Bipolar disorder is cyclical and tends to return on a somewhat regular or frequent basis. Unipolar depression also recurs, but the period between the episodes tends to be longer than with bipolar disorder. With unipolar depression, you can have a depressive episode that lasts for several months then resolves. Then you may go years without another episode.

Similarly, some people with bipolar disorder can have long inter-episode periods, but recurring episodes of depression, especially early on in your illness, tend to be suggestive of bipolar disorder.

**1 Your first depressive episode occurs before the age of 20**

The average age of onset for bipolar is 15 to 20, whereas it's 30 to 40 for unipolar depression. These are just averages, as it's possible to have your first depressive episode as a child and never develop bipolar disorder. But, generally, depression seen in bipolar disorder starts earlier than depression alone.

**2 Antidepressants sometimes don't work and can make things worse**

Antidepressants are more likely to cause mixed states where you may feel wired but tired, anxious, or agitated. You could have responded well to an

**5 You take a mood stabilizer and have a full recovery within one month**

It's tricky how important to make this sign because we use mood stabilizers as an add-on treatment for treatment-resistant depression. But the difference between the person with treatment-resistant depression and bipolar depression is in their response to an antidepressant.

## FOR THE PERSON WITH UNIPOLAR DEPRESSION

You develop depression, and your doctor prescribes an antidepressant. You have a partial response such that you feel 60%–70% better. Your doctor then adds a medication like aripiprazole (Abilify), and you notice you feel an additional 10%–20% better when taking both medications.

## FOR THE PERSON WITH BIPOLAR DEPRESSION

You develop depression symptoms, but the antidepressant doesn't help at all. In fact, you feel more agitated. You try taking another antidepressant but still don't feel well. Your doctor then adds aripiprazole, and you start to feel better but still don't feel anywhere close to your baseline. It's not until your doctor lowers

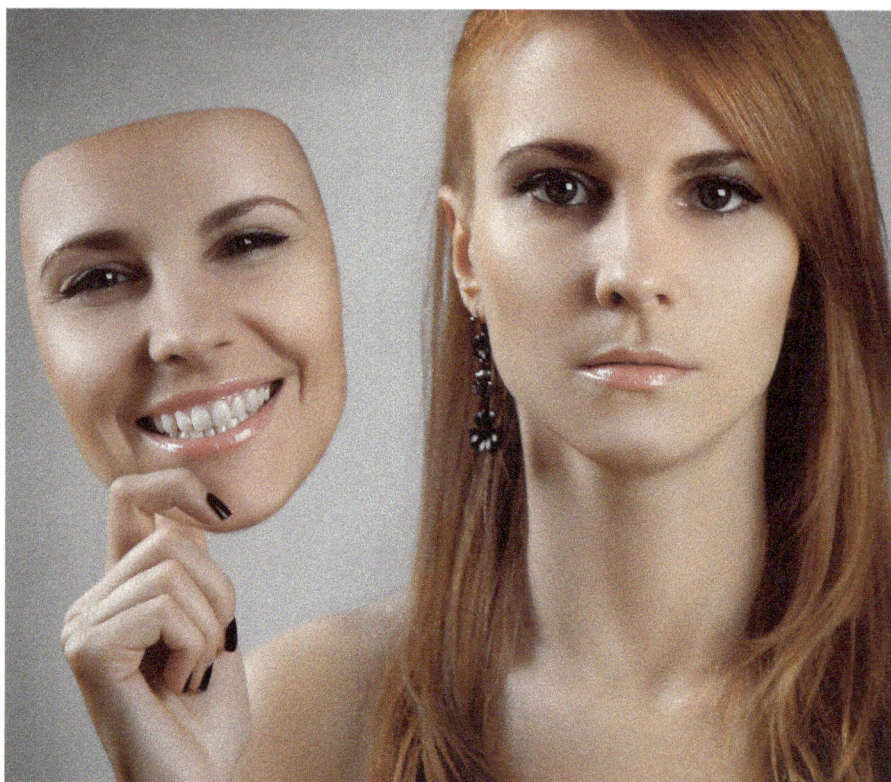

or eliminates the antidepressant that you begin to feel better.

What does it mean to be at your baseline? Your baseline is what you are like when you are neither manic or depressed. You can think of it as your "normal" self.

These are examples of how the two disorders could respond differently to the same medication combination. As with almost everything else in

life, there are no absolutes. If this has happened to you, it doesn't mean you have bipolar disorder simply because you did well on a mood stabilizer. It just means that you and your doctor should keep in mind the possibility that your depression may be part of bipolar disorder and not unipolar depression.

In the next chapter, we'll explore the differences between bipolar type 1 and bipolar type 2.

## CHAPTER 4

# Bipolar 1 vs. Bipolar 2—Which is Worse?

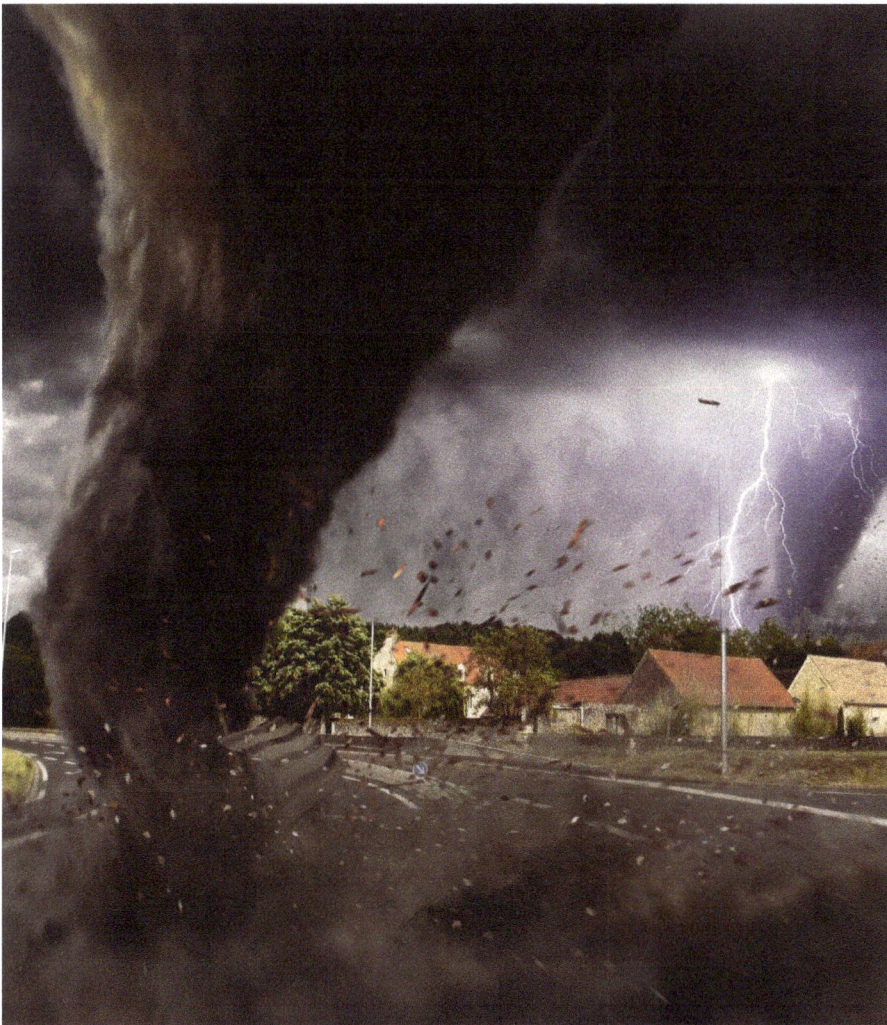

**H**ere's how the two disorders compare with each other.

Because hypomania doesn't cause as much impairment as mania, many people with bipolar 2 disorder can go their entire life without being hospitalized. By contrast, it's hard for someone with bipolar 1 to get by without ever going to the hospital. There's a good chance they will have at least one hospitalization or emergency room visit because of the degree of dysfunction caused by the mania.

Therefore, it's easy to conclude that bipolar 1 is worse than bipolar 2. A manic episode can cause a lot of destruction. It can be like a tornado ripping through your life. However, people with bipolar 2 tend to have a more

There's a common misconception that bipolar 2 disorder is a milder form of bipolar disorder. Hypomania is indeed less intense than mania. But this lesser intensity doesn't make bipolar 2 a milder illness.

A MANIC EPISODE CAN CAUSE A LOT OF DESTRUCTION. IT CAN FEEL LIKE A TORNADO RIPPING THROUGH YOUR LIFE.

chronic course to their illness. It's more chronic because they have more lifetime episodes of hypomania and depression, and the depressive episodes last longer than they do with bipolar 1. In fact, depressive episodes with bipolar 2 are more frequent and persistent than with unipolar depression.

So, in many ways, although bipolar 2 may be less intense when it comes to mania and may cause less destruction, the illness itself can create more overall dysfunction because of the lingering and recurring depressive episodes.

It's more common with bipolar 1 to have periods in between episodes (called inter-episode periods) that are longer and without symptoms. Therefore, to reduce the medication burden, some people will take a break from medication or reduce their dose during these "off" periods. This is something you should discuss with your doctor and have monitored.

But if you have bipolar 2, you're less likely to have long inter-episode periods without some depression symptoms. So, staying in treatment and addressing the chronic depressive episodes becomes even more important. A good medication regimen can help reduce the illness's overall burden by lessening symptoms and maybe even decreasing the number of recurrences you experience.

The medication you take during the maintenance phase (and when it would be appropriate to take a break) will be addressed in Chapter 18.

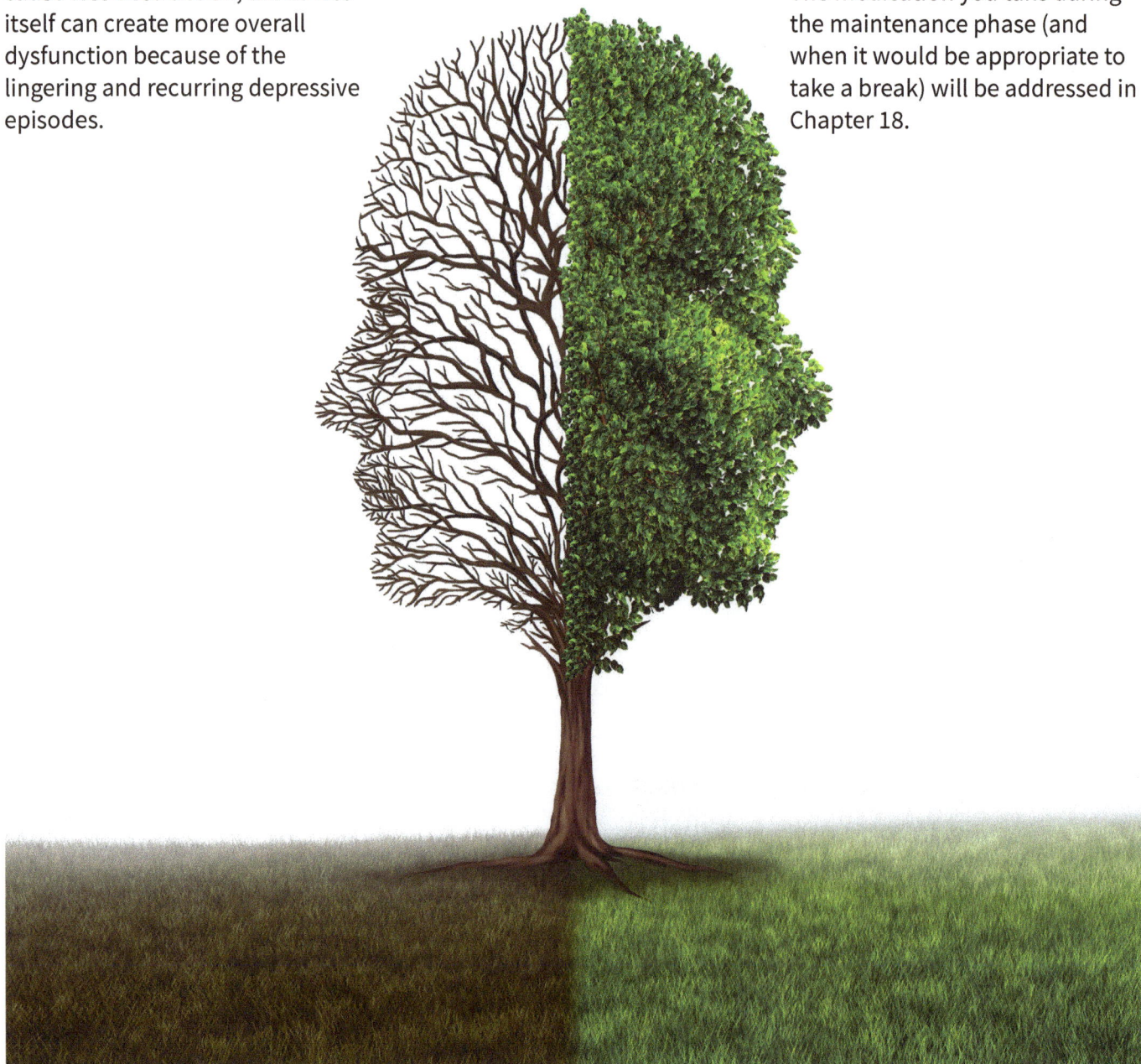

## CHAPTER 5

# What is Bipolar Spectrum?

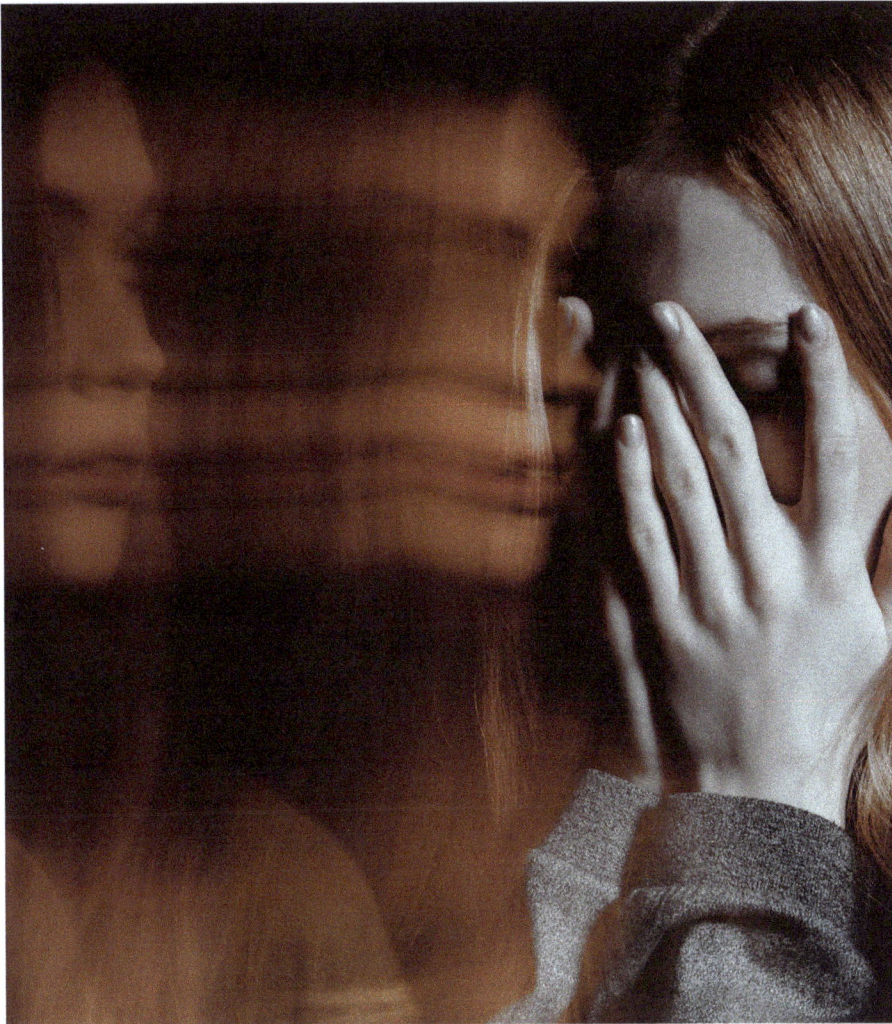

**T**his concept of a bipolar spectrum dates back to the early 1900s and Emil Kraepelin, a German psychiatrist.

Dr. Kraepelin is considered the father of modern psychiatry. He identified and defined schizophrenia and manic depression, which he termed manic-depressive insanity in his book, *Manic-Depressive Insanity and Paranoia*, first published in 1921. This is where we get the now obsolete term, manic depression.

Manic-depressive insanity was a recurring illness of both depression and mania, with or without psychosis. The illness's key feature was that it was episodic, and episodes would come and go.

In the United States, "bipolar spectrum" is not an official term. However, whether bipolar disorder and depression should be considered a unified bipolar spectrum illness is being debated among experts in the field.

{ THE KEY FEATURE OF MANIC DEPRESSION IS RECURRENT EPISODES OF EITHER DEPRESSION OR MANIA. }

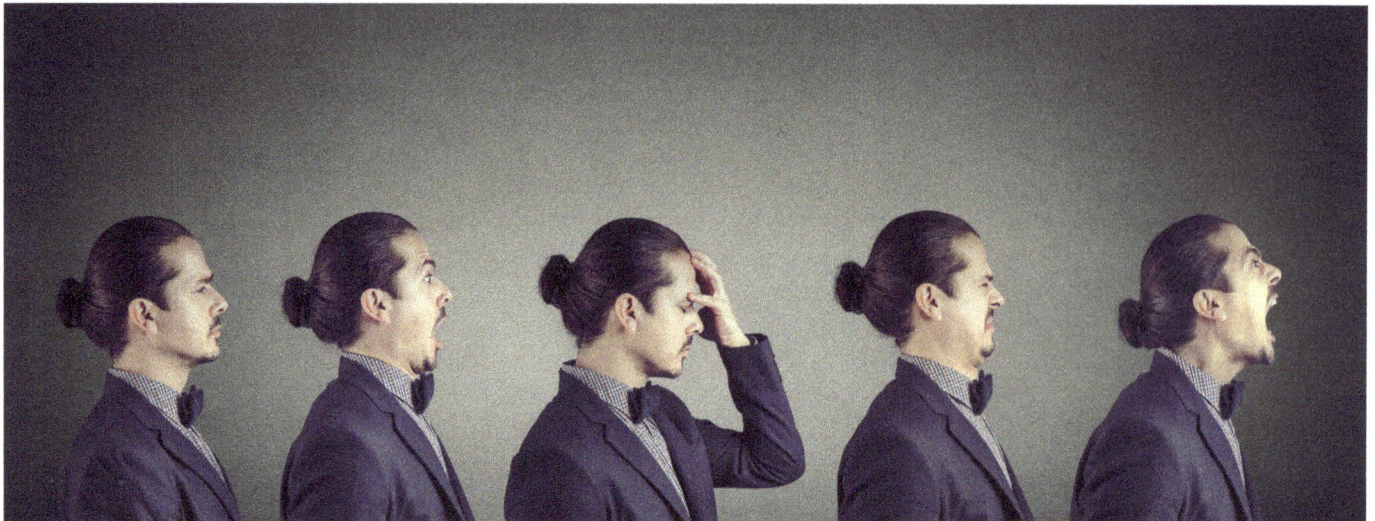

This is different from other psychiatric illnesses. With schizophrenia, once the illness appears, it remains. The symptoms may wax and wane in intensity, but they're always present to some degree.

People with anxiety can have waves of it where the anxiety is intense and unmanageable and, some time later, it improves. But they still have some degree of anxiety that's always present but manageable. Since anxiety disorders are lifelong, you may see this as usual for you. You may believe that things bother you more than other people, and it's not a big deal.

**SOME PEOPLE BELIEVE THE ORIGINAL CONCEPT OF MANIC DEPRESSION BETTER FITS WHAT CLINICIANS SEE IN PRACTICE.**

With attention deficit hyperactivity disorder (ADHD), the peak occurrence of the illness is in childhood. Like anxiety, it can completely resolve or improve to the point where symptoms are manageable. Many people continue to have symptoms as adults.

But depression and mania act differently. The manic or depressive episodes can quickly surface and then quickly resolve. Sometimes depression, however, can last for an extended period, spanning even years. But for the most part, the nature of mood disorders is that depression and mania come and go, with periods of being close or back to your baseline in between episodes.

This is how Dr. Kraepelin conceptualized this illness. He called it manic depression. The insanity part comes with psychosis occurring in either the manic state or the depressive state.

In 1980 the third edition of the *Diagnostic Statistical Manual of*

*Mental Disorders* was published, and manic-depressive insanity was split into bipolar disorder and unipolar major depression. With this change, the key feature of the illness became polarity rather than episodes.

So, it was thought that the experience of having opposite disordered mood states is a separate phenomenon from having the same mood state that repeats. Therefore, repeating episodes of depression was carved out as a distinct illness called major depression. Experiencing repeating episodes of opposite poles of mania and depression was assigned to a separate diagnostic category: bipolar disorder.

Not everyone accepted this change. Some believed that Dr. Kraepelin's original broader concept of manic depression more accurately described what clinicians see in practice. Some researchers concluded that there is more to bipolar disorder than just mania and depression, and we should change the term to bipolar spectrum to include other conditions like:

- Recurrent severe depression with psychosis
- Depression, with mixed symptoms
- Cyclothymia (see chapter 6)
- Antidepressant-induced mania
- Anxious depression
- Atypical depression.

Atypical depression is a subtype of major depression with specific features like increased appetite, increased sleep, and having positive experiences improve your mood transiently.

Usually, having a good day doesn't brighten up your mood when you have depression. In fact, one of the symptoms of depression is anhedonia. Anhedonia is when you're unable to find joy or pleasure in anything.

Some go further and believe that depression doesn't occur without mania. This concept is called the primacy of mania. However, this viewpoint is not as popular and accepted as the view of mania and depression being grouped together as a single bipolar spectrum illness.

## WHAT'S THE PRACTICAL APPLICATION OF THE BIPOLAR SPECTRUM ISSUE?

Some people with depression worry that their doctor may have missed their "real" diagnosis of bipolar disorder.

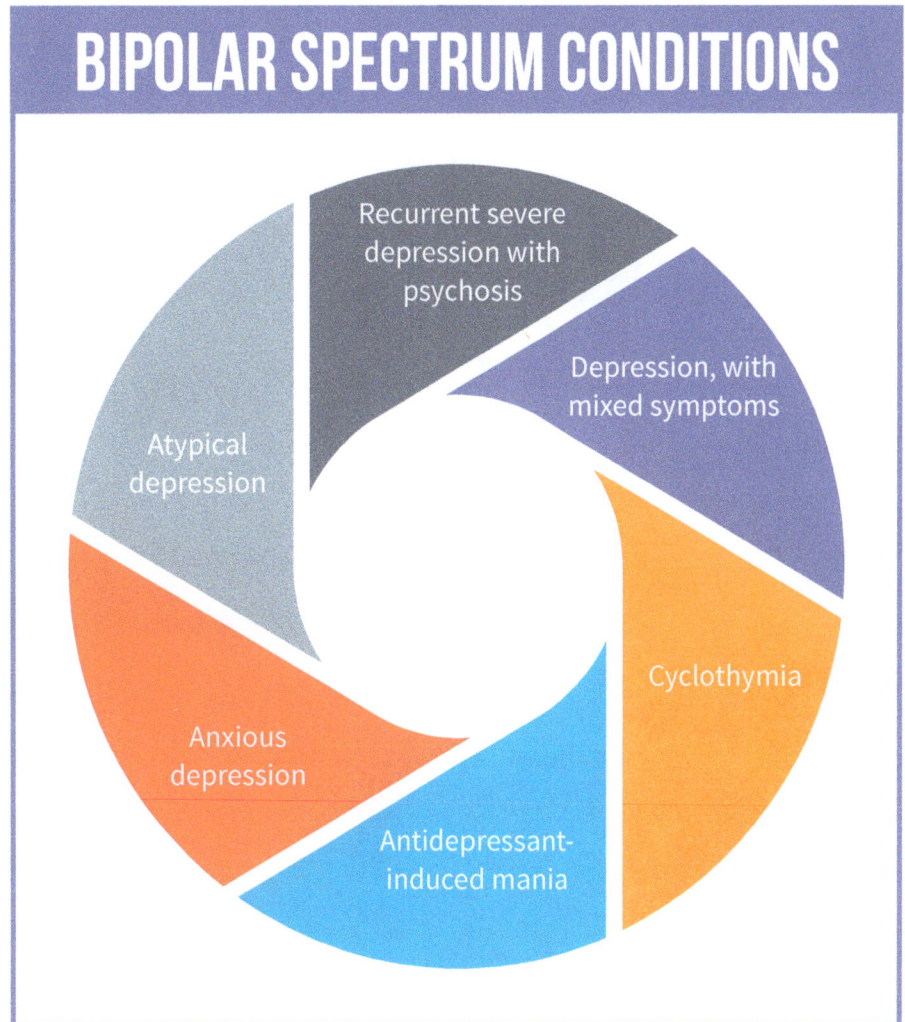

BIPOLAR SPECTRUM CONDITIONS

Recurrent severe depression with psychosis

Depression, with mixed symptoms

Cyclothymia

Antidepressant-induced mania

Anxious depression

Atypical depression

If we changed the disorder to a bipolar spectrum illness, one end of the spectrum would be depression alone. The other end would be a combination of depression and mania/hypomania. A person can remain at the depression end of the spectrum without ever developing mania or hypomania. Not everyone on the spectrum would necessarily experience anxious symptoms or hypomania.

Suppose you have a first-degree relative with bipolar disorder, such as a parent or sibling. In that case, you have a greater risk of manifesting mania or hypomania

at some point, but it's still not a given.

Therefore, if you've only had depression and no mania, you would still be treated with an antidepressant first until there's a clear reason to add a mood stabilizer. Reasons to add a mood stabilizer would be emerging mania or hypomania, or if your depression didn't respond adequately to a mood stabilizer alone. This is known as treatment-resistant depression. The treatment for treatment-resistant depression is similar to the treatment for bipolar disorder.

## CHAPTER 6

# How Is Cyclothymia Different From Bipolar Disorder?

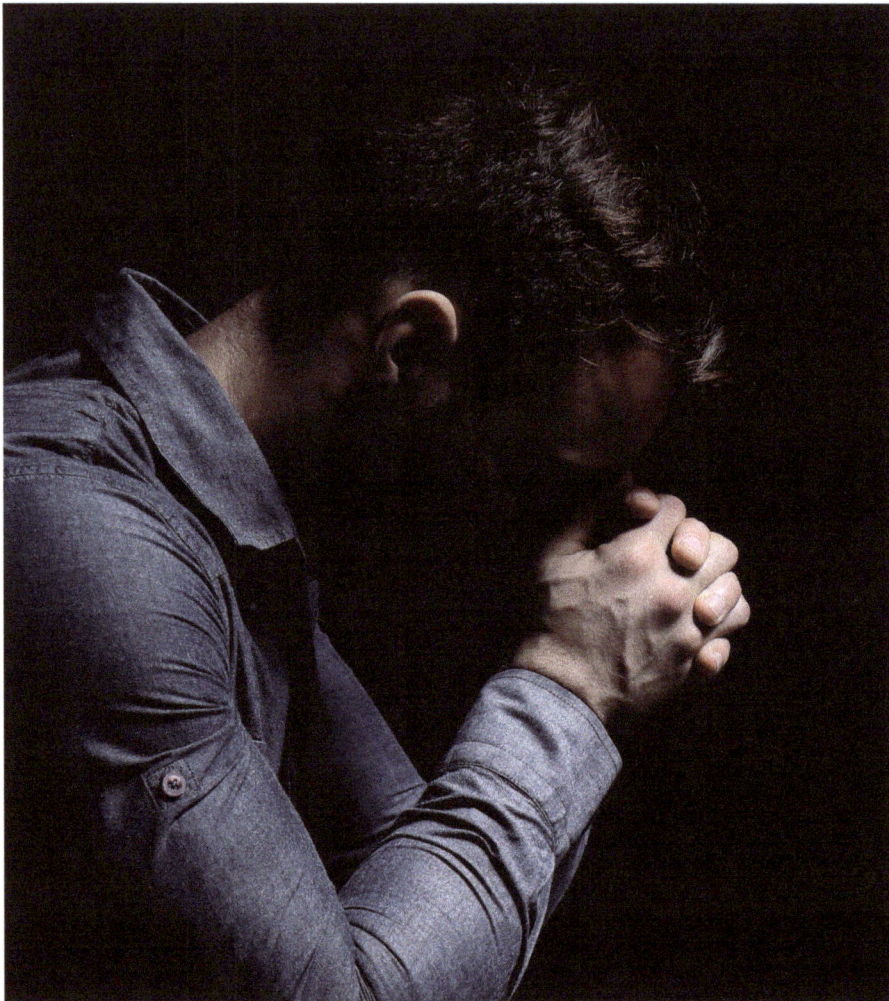

With cyclothymia, you have hypomanic symptoms but not enough to be considered a full hypomanic episode. You also have symptoms of depression but not enough to be considered a full depressive episode. So, it's like having subthreshold hypomania and subthreshold depression.

Here are the symptoms of a hypomanic episode (they are the same as mania):

1 Decreased need for sleep (such as feeling rested after only 3 hours of sleep).
2 More talkative than usual or pressure to keep talking.
3 Racing thoughts.
4 Distractibility.

Cyclothymia is very similar to bipolar 2. With bipolar 2, you have episodes of hypomania and episodes of depression.

{ **15%–20%** OF PEOPLE WITH CYCLOTHYMIA DEVELOP BIPOLAR DISORDER. }

**5** Increase in agitation or goal-directed activity. This can include hypersexuality or excessive involvement in activities with a high potential for painful consequences (e.g., buying sprees, sexual indiscretions, foolish business investments, etc.).

**6** Inflated self-esteem or grandiosity.

**7** Excessive involvement in risky activities with the potential for painful consequences.

With bipolar 2 disorder, you need three or four of these symptoms. But with cyclothymia, you may only have one to two symptoms.

There are nine symptoms of a depressive episode:

**1** Depressed mood most of the day

**2** Very little interest in pleasurable activities

**3** Weight changes

**4** Sleep changes

**5** Being physically slow or agitated

**6** Fatigue or energy loss

**7** Feelings of worthlessness or guilt

**8** Problems with thinking or concentration

**9** Recurrent thoughts of death or feeling suicidal.

For a depressive episode, you need to have five of nine of these symptoms. With cyclothymia, you could have one to five. With

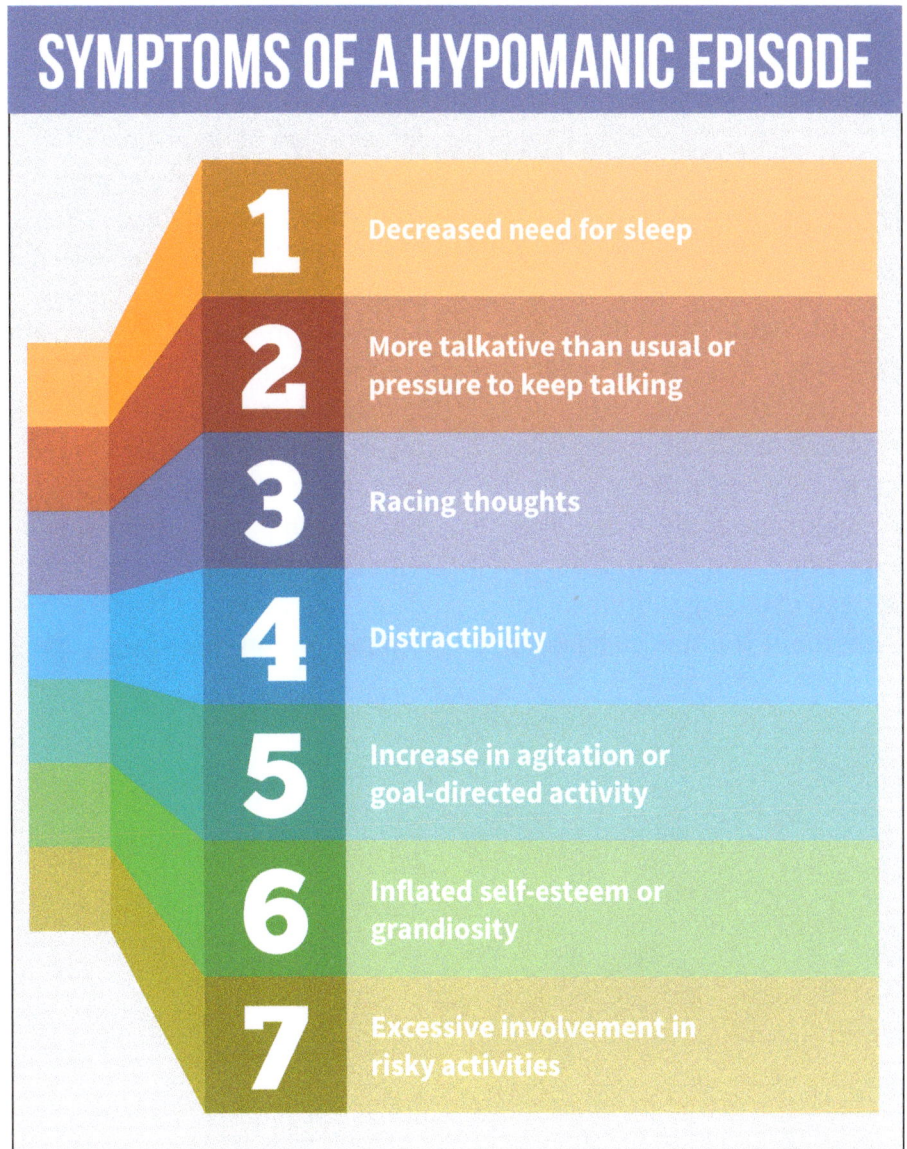

## SYMPTOMS OF A HYPOMANIC EPISODE

**1** Decreased need for sleep

**2** More talkative than usual or pressure to keep talking

**3** Racing thoughts

**4** Distractibility

**5** Increase in agitation or goal-directed activity

**6** Inflated self-esteem or grandiosity

**7** Excessive involvement in risky activities

bipolar 2, your episodes of either depression or hypomania need to last at least four days. But with cyclothymia, either of the states lasts less than four days.

Even though you don't need that many symptoms of either state, you need a pattern of these up and down mood states that lasts for at least two years. So cyclothymia is a chronic disorder of fluctuating moods.

With bipolar disorder, you can have inter-episode periods lasting months to years. With

cyclothymic disorder, the period in between states lasts no more than two months. This means that, most of the time, you're having symptoms of one state or the other. Cyclothymic disorder behaves similarly to bipolar disorder, with rapid cycling. Rapid cycling will be addressed in Chapter 7.

## WHEN DOES IT START?

Cyclothymic disorder usually starts in adolescence or early adulthood. It is sometimes present in children, and the mean age of onset for the child version is six.

## DOES IT ALWAYS TURN INTO BIPOLAR DISORDER?

Cyclothymic disorder doesn't necessarily convert to bipolar disorder, but it's estimated that 15% to 50% of people with cyclothymic disorder go on to develop bipolar disorder, either type 1 or 2. This means that, instead of having subthreshold symptoms, you start to have full hypomanic, manic, or depressive symptoms.

Some researchers consider cyclothymic disorder as more of a temperament issue or disorder of development. You may see internet articles calling it a cyclothymic disposition or cyclothymic temperament. This would be another way of describing a person with a moody personality. People would see them as generally moody. The reason for considering it part of your temperament is that the symptoms aren't severe enough to cause the same problems as bipolar disorder, and they can seem like they're just part of your personality.

We typically don't treat cyclothymia with medication because the symptoms usually aren't severe enough. You should always weigh the risks and benefits of medications. Medications come with potential side effects to which you may not want to be exposed, especially if you can overcome your symptoms with therapy.

## CHAPTER 7

# Rapid Cycling Bipolar and Mixed Features

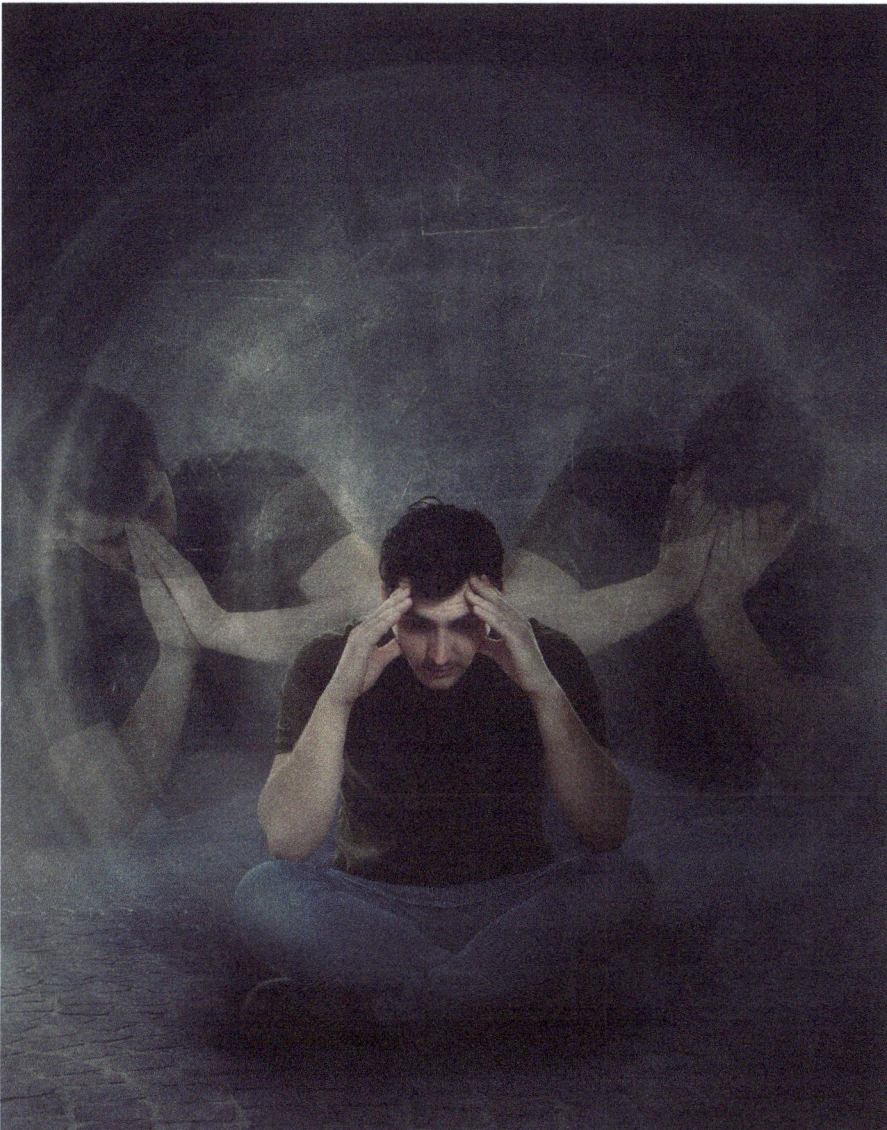

## RAPID CYCLING

With bipolar disorder, the duration of episode is two weeks for depression, one week for mania, and four days for hypomania. These are minimum amounts of time, and these episodes can last longer. In fact, depression usually lasts several months, if not longer.

If you have more than four episodes of either depression or mania/hypomania in a year, you're considered to have a rapid cycling form of bipolar disorder. Rapid cycling is called a course specifier. It's not a separate diagnosis; instead, it's a description added to the end of the diagnosis to give more details about how the illness manifests. If you had more than four episodes in a year, your diagnosis would be

This chapter addresses two variations in bipolar disorder: rapid cycling and mixed features.

SHIFTING EMOTIONS IS NOT THE SAME AS SHIFTING AN ENTIRE MOOD STATE, SUCH AS THE SHIFT FROM MANIA TO DEPRESSION.

bipolar 1 or bipolar 2, with rapid cycling.

Rapid cycling bipolar occurs in about 10–15% of people with bipolar disorder. We tend to see it more with bipolar 2 than bipolar 1.

Ultra-rapid cycling is not an official term in our diagnostic manual. It's a term that researchers have coined and use to give an even more detailed description of how the illness behaves. People call it ultra-rapid cycling when a person has mood switches each month and ultra-ultra-rapid cycling, also called ultradian, when a person has mood cycles lasting a day.

This definition doesn't align with the *DSM-5* description of the mood episodes. According to the *DSM*, the shortest episode that you can have is 4 days for hypomania. One day of symptoms wouldn't be considered a full hypomanic episode. This is why using this term is controversial and it hasn't been officially adopted.

It's important to tell the difference between shifting emotions and shifting a complete mood state. Your mood is how you feel emotionally. Your mood state, such as depression or mania, refers to a group of symptoms, including your activity level, sleep, and motivation. In a depressed state, you tend to be slowed down in many ways, and with mania, you're sped up in many ways.

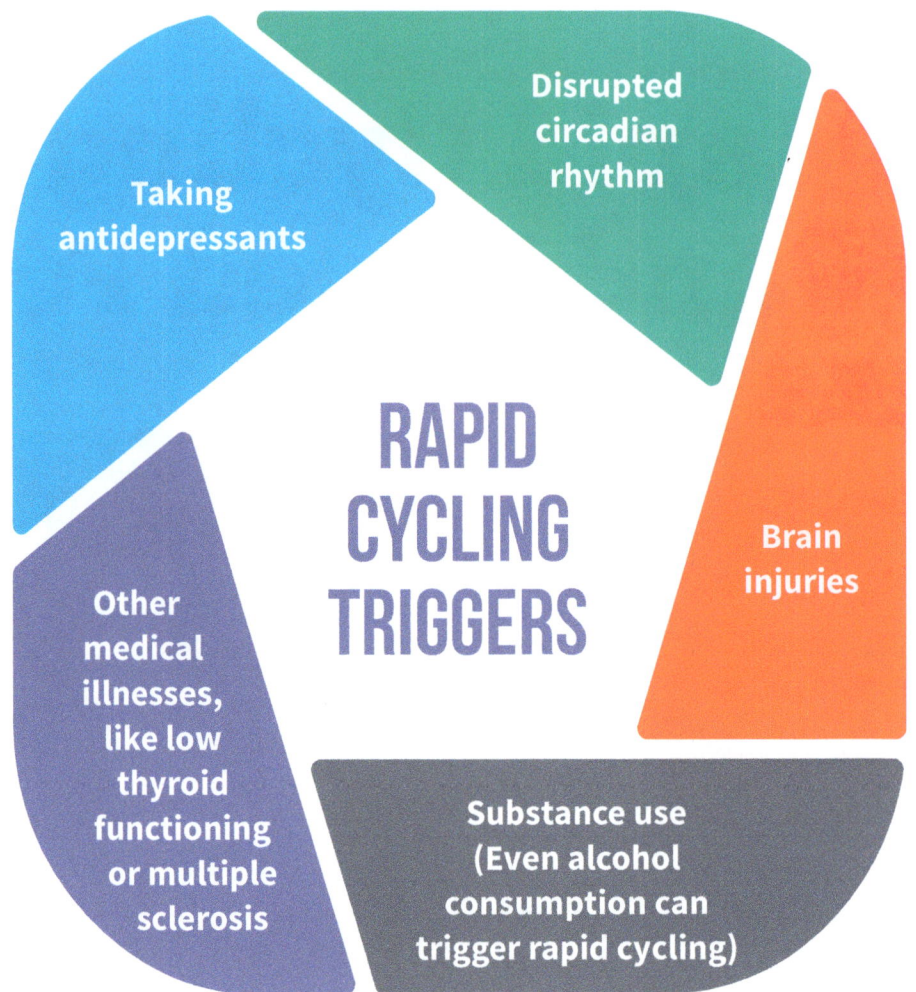

**RAPID CYCLING TRIGGERS**

- Taking antidepressants
- Disrupted circadian rhythm
- Brain injuries
- Substance use (Even alcohol consumption can trigger rapid cycling)
- Other medical illnesses, like low thyroid functioning or multiple sclerosis

So, with rapid cycling, you'll go from feeling sped up to feeling slowed down and go back and forth between these states. That's not the same as switching from crying to laughing over a day. That would be an emotional change, not necessarily a mood state change. This emotional lability is only one aspect of bipolar disorder. There's more to bipolar disorder than shifting emotions.

Emotional changes can also happen with borderline personality disorder or post-traumatic stress disorder (PTSD).

But let's say you do have ultra-rapid cycling with true switching of mood states that occurs monthly. Why would this happen?

Some things can destabilize bipolar disorder and make you switch states more frequently. These include:

- A disrupted circadian rhythm that results in an irregular sleep or eating schedule.

An example of this would be nearly reversing your day-night schedule such that you're sleeping most of the day and sleeping very little during the night. People with bipolar disorder are sensitive to biological rhythms. Getting off track with these basic routines can trigger a relapse of an episode or cause you to switch back and forth between episodes (e.g., going from mania to depression or vice versa). Working night shifts can also make this happen.

- Brain injuries. This doesn't have to be the kind of head injury secondary to a gunshot wound or falling from a roof and losing consciousness. The brain has a very soft consistency and floats in your skull surrounded by fluid. Your skull protects it, but you can get a brain injury like a concussion from being knocked around or hit in the head. This kind of head trauma can result in mood changes. Having a stroke can produce similar mood changes.
- Substance use (even alcohol consumption can trigger rapid cycling).
- Other medical illnesses, like low thyroid functioning or multiple sclerosis.
- Taking antidepressants.

It's generally recommended to minimize antidepressant use for treating bipolar disorder because some studies show that antidepressants can trigger mood switching or rapid cycling. It doesn't happen to everyone. But if you have rapid cycling symptoms, you should avoid antidepressants.

## MIXED FEATURES

With bipolar disorder, you can have episodes of hypomania or mania and depression. Sometimes you may experience both of these states at the same time. We call these mixed episodes. The official term is bipolar disorder, either 1 or 2, with mixed features.

For example, you may have a depressed mood occasioned by crying spells, yet your mind is racing and you're aggravated. You may be making impulsive decisions yet have trouble getting motivated to get out of bed in the mornings.

It's like you're a hyped-up, sad or negative person. It can feel extremely uncomfortable. Bipolar disorder with mixed features is harder to treat than bipolar disorder alone.

Not all of the medications used to treat bipolar disorder also work for mixed episodes. Medication options for the different phases of bipolar disorder will be addressed in Chapter 16. But be prepared: mixed features are harder to treat, and there's a good chance you'll need to take more than one medication at the same time. Generally, taking an antidepressant for mixed mania is discouraged.

## WHAT IF THE MEDICATION DOESN'T WORK?

If you can't get well with medication, another solution to consider is electroconvulsive therapy (ECT). ECT works by provoking a seizure under tightly controlled conditions. Your body doesn't convulse when under anesthesia. But your brain is still stimulated. Stimulating the brain in this manner treats many conditions, including depression, mania, and psychosis. ECT has been used in psychiatry since the 1930s and continues to be the gold standard treatment for conditions that are nonresponsive to medication.

Transcranial magnetic stimulation (TMS) stimulates the brain without producing a seizure. It uses an electromagnetic field to stimulate the dorsolateral prefrontal cortex, which is a part of the brain involved in mood regulation. TMS is approved by the United States Food and Drug Administration (FDA) for treatment-resistant (unipolar) depression. In early 2020 the FDA granted breakthrough device designation to one company to develop a protocol for using TMS for bipolar depression.

These heavy-duty treatments are highly effective but require significant commitment and careful monitoring. Other non-medication treatments will be addressed in Chapters 19 and 20.

> **WITH MIXED FEATURES YOU EXPERIENCE MANIA AND DEPRESSION SIMULTANEOUSLY.**

## CHAPTER 8

# How Mania Drives Your Sexuality

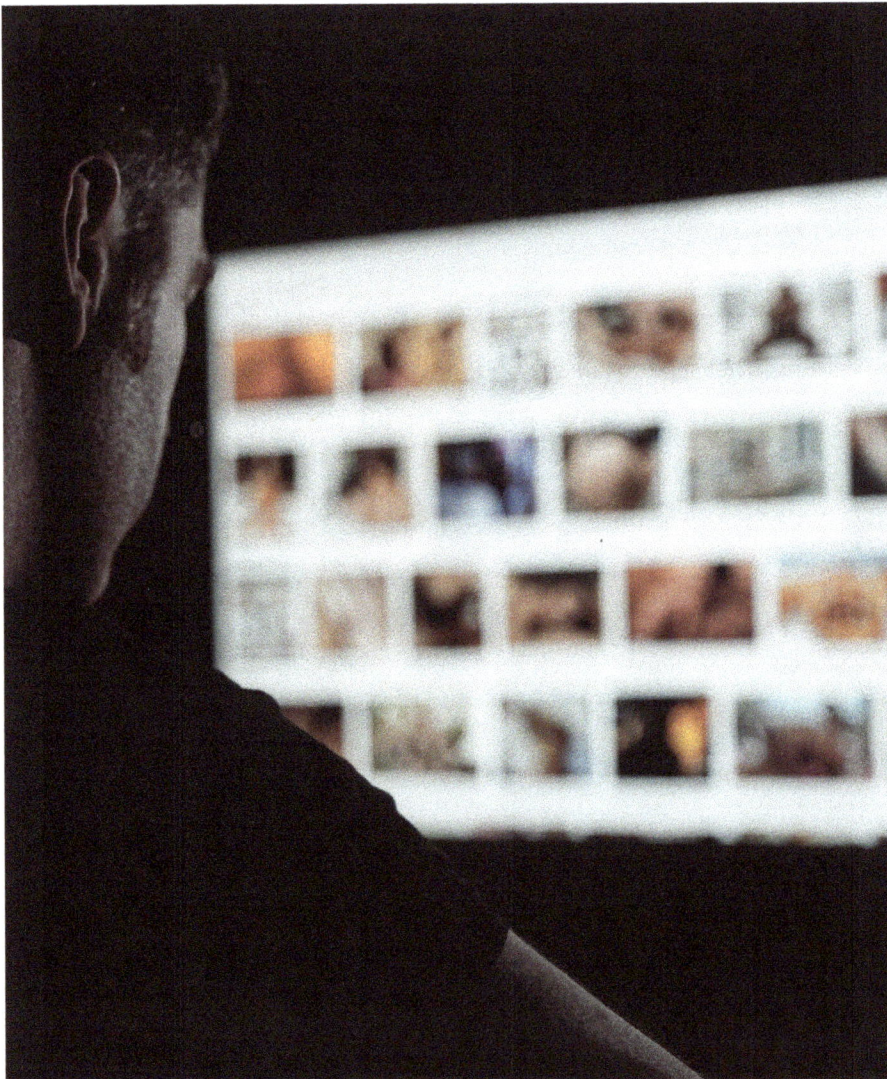

For the remainder of the discussion, I will use "mania" and "hypomania" interchangeably.

Being manic is like a car engine idling high. Everything moves faster, including your thoughts and impulses. This affects your judgment and decision making. Your sexuality is a core part of your identity and is a basic, primal need. Everyone has some degree of sexual desire. You may suppress it because of social conventions and expectations, but it's a part of our makeup that's always present. It's similar to your primary desire to attach to someone. Everyone has that need to some degree. Some need attachment more than others.

When you become manic and your engine is turned up,

Hypersexuality is one of the symptoms associated with the manic or hypomanic phase of bipolar disorder. It falls under the category of increased goal-directed activity.

YOUR SEXUALITY IS A CORE PART OF YOUR IDENTITY AND IS A PRIMARY NEED.

these primal needs and desires increase. You have an increased appetite for many things, not just sex. If you combine this increased appetite with fast-moving thoughts, poor impulse control, and poor insight and judgment, what do you get? You get unrestrained gratification seeking.

There are different ways this gratification seeking can look.

Here's an example. Bob decides to start a new company that solves a unique problem that no one else can solve. He withdraws all of his savings and invests it into a process that will kick-start his company. Bob is convinced this new company will change the industry as no other company has to date. He goes several nights without sleeping to work on the launch because, in his mind, the country really needs this right now.

Here's another one. Shirley has the urge to speak to her best friend, Julie, who's working. But Shirley really needs to speak to Julie right away. So, she has Julie pulled out of a meeting to talk with her. Shirley just wants to tell Julie how much she values their friendship. Shirley feels much relief after letting Julie know her feelings.

Can you imagine how these two people may be feeling with their sense of urgency and poor judgment?

With hypersexuality, you start with your basic sexual need

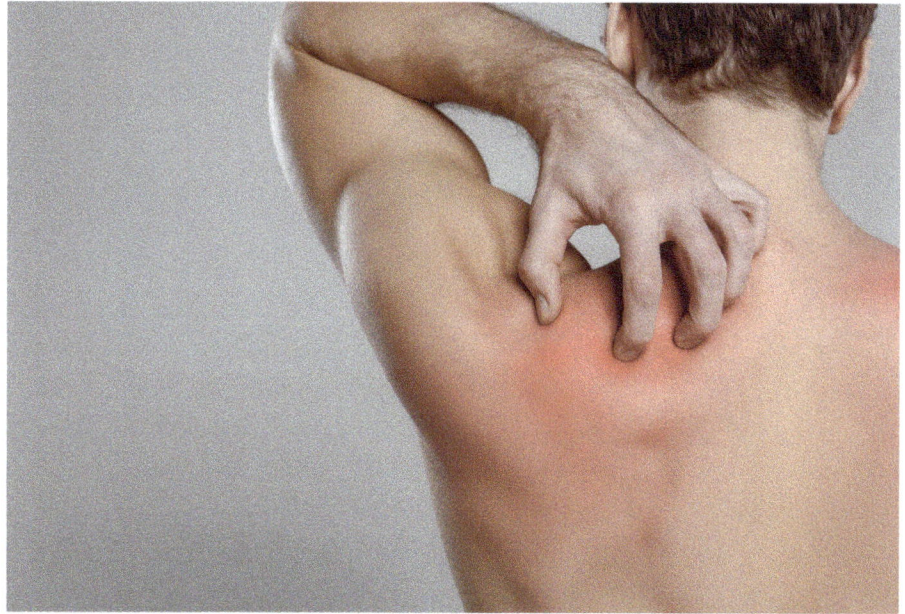

and add increased energy around it in a way that creates an uncontrollable urge. It's like having an itch in the middle of your back that you can't reach. You find something with which to scratch the itch, and feel some relief, initially. But there's still one area you can't find, and it's still itching. You find yourself scratching all around your back, but that spot is still itching.

This itching analogy is similar to hypersexuality because the scratching feels good, but you're also over-scratching parts of your body. So, the inability to completely satisfy the itch is unsatisfying, and, in the end, the result is you feel good and bad simultaneously.

From the perspective of a person not affected by mania, it may seem like the manic person is just having fun and being self-indulgent. But it's not all fun. For many, it just doesn't feel that good, or it yields temporary satisfaction.

Many people will feel shame when the mania resolves because, unlike a sexual addiction, hypersexuality in mania is only present during the manic or hypomanic episode. After that passes, you return to your usual behavior. What's more, often with bipolar disorder, the opposite mood follows. The mania will be followed by depression either immediately or some time later. If a person who was hypersexual while they were manic then gets depressed, their sex drive is shot, and they become hypersexual. In fact, this may be a period of mourning the losses and damage they created during the mania.

## WHAT ARE SOME HYPERSEXUAL BEHAVIORS?

They can include increased sexual activity either with your partner or multiple partners, or even with strangers. A person who would otherwise never consider being unfaithful could have an affair during this period, not only because of the increased urges they feel but also because of poor judgment, trouble controlling impulses, and misperception of their world and what's going on around them. They can get tunnel vision. Nothing else exists except them and the other person or people.

But not everyone has sex with multiple partners. Some people masturbate excessively. Masturbation is considered a normal activity, but some people will lose track of time watching pornography and masturbating all day.

Another more subtle presentation is getting lost in sexual fantasies. This could look like daydreaming about sexual acts to the extent that you lose track of time, neglect other responsibilities, or get distracted from work or school.

## WHAT CAN YOU DO ABOUT THIS?

The immediate solution is to treat the episode. As I mentioned, if the hypersexuality is from mania and not from a sexual disorder, the hypersexuality resolves when the mania resolves. You don't become nonsexual. Your baseline sexuality returns.

If you have a partner and you're having an affair during an episode, you should have a couples therapy session to help you and your partner understand what happened. Then, the burden is on you to keep yourself well and continue to look for the early signs of your mania so that you don't repeat the same behavior.

In the throes of a manic episode, your judgment disappears, and it's easy to forget the damage caused by the last episode. It's like being in the movie *Groundhog Day*, where the main character becomes stuck in a loop, and the day repeats itself over and over again. If you're not proactive, each manic episode could feel like another day repeating itself. And you may be able to deal with the consequences, but the people your behavior affects may eventually give up on you and abandon the relationship.

## CHAPTER 9

# The Manic Prodrome –Three Signs Your Mania is Coming

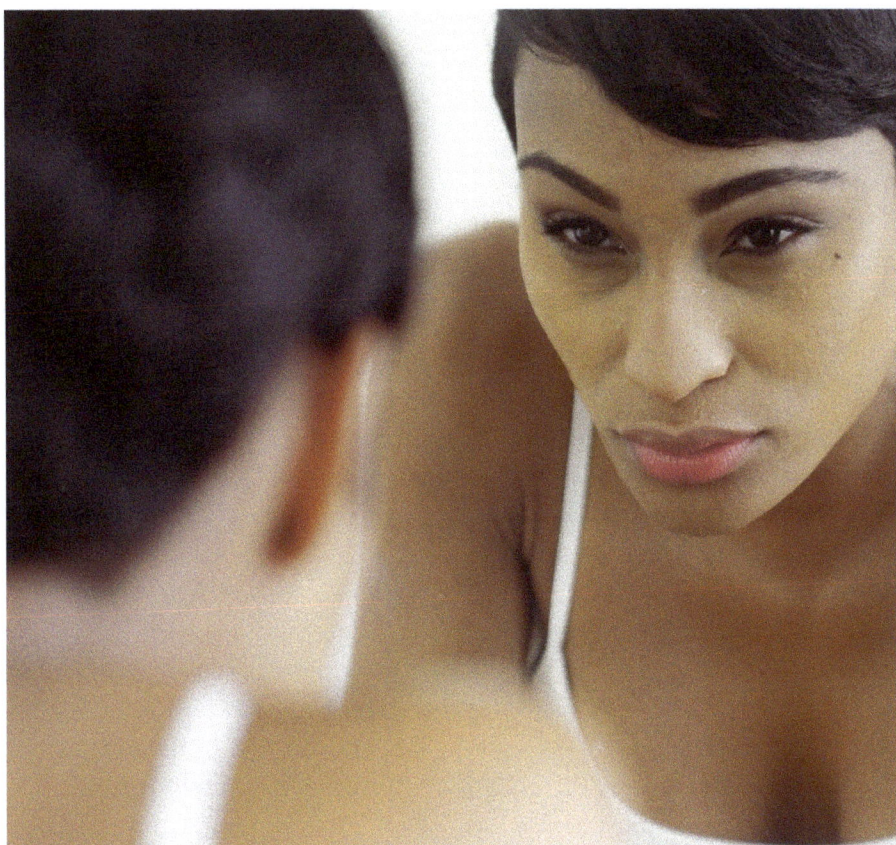

**E**ven if you can't stop the hurricane, you can brace for it by boarding up the windows and stocking up on water.

Similarly, bipolar disorder is progressive. The episodes build momentum. The prodrome is the period of milder symptoms that precede the more severe symptoms. This period can last for weeks to months. With bipolar disorder, you can have a prodromal period before depression as well as before the mania.

The most common prodromal symptoms for mania tend to be an elevated mood, decreased

What are the early signs that you're about to have a manic episode? We call these early signs the prodrome. Being able to detect early signs of a manic episode can be helpful in either preventing the episode or lessening its impact. It's like preparing for a hurricane.

THE PRODROME IS THE PERIOD OF MILDER SYMPTOMS THAT PRECEDE THE MORE SEVERE SYMPTOMS.

need for sleep, and increased activity. These symptoms can build for several weeks before they get out of control, or evolve to where you have a manic or hypomanic episode.

Let's look more closely at these symptoms.

## ELEVATED MOOD

One of the problems with the manic phase is that you usually don't see the early symptoms as a problem. It will often take someone close to you to recognize that your mood is elevated beyond what someone would normally expect. But even with this recognition, it still may be hard to notice this particular symptom. But remember, this is more than just feeling great. It may be feeling invincible or having way more confidence and audacity than you usually do. It's something that stands out in some way.

## DECREASED NEED FOR SLEEP

Needing less sleep is usually easier to recognize than a lift in your mood. Needing less sleep is different from disrupted or choppy sleep. With bipolar disorder, even when you are between episodes, you can still have poor quality sleep. Examples of this would be taking longer to fall asleep or not being able to sleep straight through the night. Sometimes between episodes, you can have day-night reversal such that you can't go to sleep until the early hours of the morning. Then you're sleeping

most of the day and up most of the night.

However, in the prodrome phase, you don't need as much sleep to feel rested. You may be oblivious to the fact that it's time to go to bed. You may stay up doing things during the night because you're not tired. If this happens, an early intervention could be to see your doctor and make medication adjustments, like increasing your mood stabilizer. It could mean stopping taking an antidepressant you were on because of a previous depressive episode. Or your doctor could add a medication to help you sleep. These adjustments could halt the mania's progression or lessen the episode's severity.

## INCREASED ACTIVITY

Hypersexuality is an example of increased activity. Another example is becoming more involved in your job and working more hours. If you're a student, you could have more energy to study for longer.

Here's an example. Jane has bipolar disorder and is a musician. Jane recognized that an early sign that she's becoming manic is when she starts creating music tracks in her mind. This may sound like a good thing because, after all, she's a musician. But her talent consists of playing an instrument, not writing music. It was only when she became manic that she spent time in her head developing musical scores. Then when she was out of the episode, she

thought the music she created was terrible. So, it's not as if the mania was a wonderfully creative time for her to extend her skills to writing music. Instead, it was an unproductive musical exploration that never resulted in anything usable. So, Jane knew that whenever she began to write music in her head, she needed to call her doctor.

People in this phase may also feel like they need to move around. This is called agitation. It can take the form of pacing, not being able to sit still, or feeling markedly impatient. If left unchecked, the agitation can evolve into irritability or aggression.

Early in your illness, you probably won't recognize these signs. It's only in retrospect that you can look back and see the buildup. In fact, even after multiple episodes, you may still have trouble seeing the symptoms as they play out.

Here's an approach that may help. After you have recovered from your last episode and are in between episodes, look back at what happened in the weeks or months leading up to your most

> YOU PROBABLY WON'T RECOGNIZE THE SIGNS EARLY IN YOUR ILLNESS. IT MAY TAKE A FEW EPISODES TO SEE THE PATTERN.

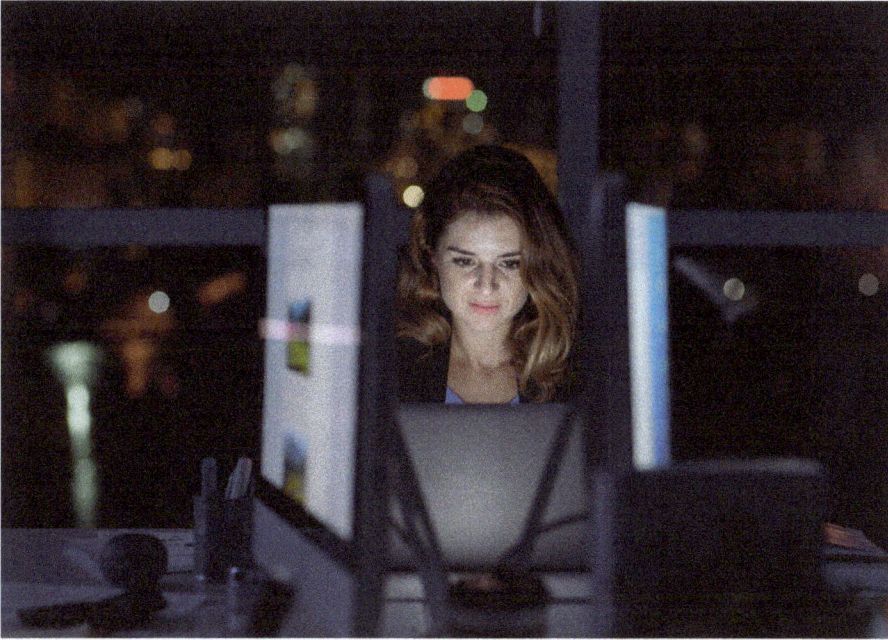

especially if your sleep is undisturbed. But it's still helpful to be on alert because things can change rapidly with bipolar disorder.

If you don't have a regular sleep schedule, this is one of the first things to change. People with bipolar disorder are highly sensitive to changes in routine. It's been shown that sticking to a regular routine, where you do certain things around the same time every day, shortens the recovery time from an episode and lengthens the time between episodes. You will learn more about Social Rhythm Therapy in Chapter 19.

Another reason to have a regular sleep schedule is to track when you're sleeping less. Adults need an average of 7–9 hours of sleep. Many people with bipolar disorder have trouble sleeping more than 6 hours. But that should be the minimum amount for you to aim at. Sleeping less than 6 hours sets you up for problems such as triggering rapid cycling of your episodes.

recent episode. Can you recognize any of the symptoms from these three categories that fit you? Is there something on which you tend to hyper-focus? This could be an increased sexual desire. It could also be your involvement in a group or club for which you usually don't have time.  But when you start getting manic, you re-engage with this entity and become super-involved.

These are general examples to help you self-reflect. Take a hard look at your behavior and try to identify patterns. You may need your doctor, therapist, or a close friend to help you see the patterns. Then write down the behavior and let someone close to you know what you do so they can help you recognize early signs.

If you see mania or hypomania returning, you should visit your doctor for a follow-up appointment. You may not need a change in your medication,

## CHAPTER 10

# Can Working Too Intensely Make You Manic?

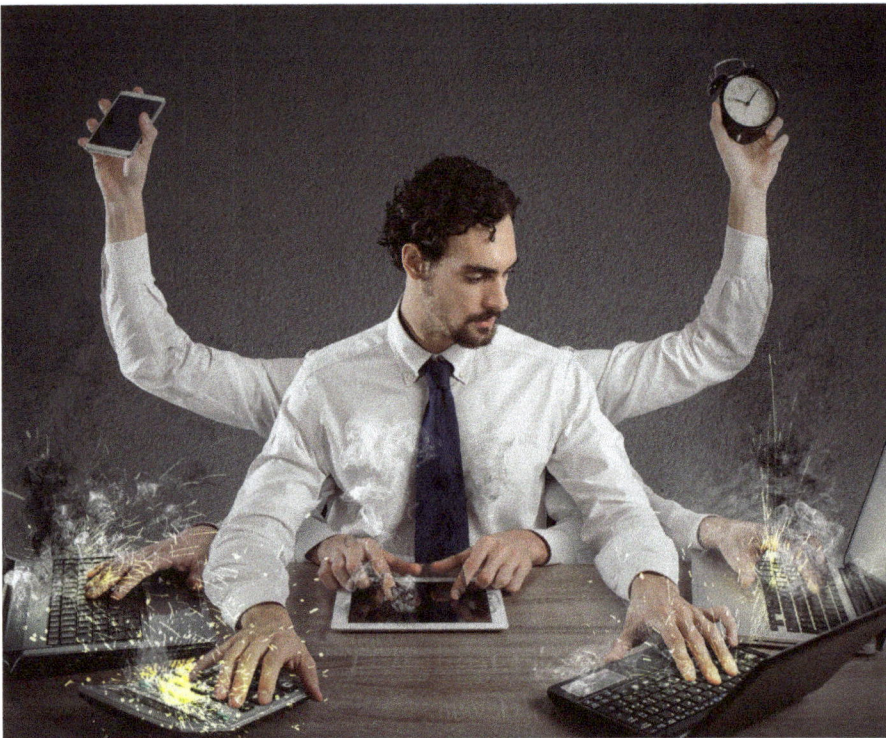

This chapter is based on a question from a viewer of my YouTube channel. The question is shortened and paraphrased in certain parts. Here's the gist. Judy feels she can't do the things she used to do because of her bipolar illness. Essentially, she feels held back because she fears that working hard will trigger a manic episode.

Here's Judy's question.

*For YEARS I built my life into developing myself into a media mogul focusing on eco-conscious innovators and entrepreneurs, and for a very short time I had great success, including having a public-access/cable TV show with several pilot episodes and a number of websites that I was building up with online courses, networking events, and other social media platforms. Over the years, my involvement in building this "business" took a toll on my marriage, leading to divorce, and put a strain on my family. This is mainly because they didn't believe I'd be successful and thought I should get a "real job."*

*I had my first manic episode, at which time I was hospitalized, and at that time, I got my official diagnosis of bipolar 1. I was 35 at this time. Now that I am stable and medicated, I'm afraid of stepping back into the limelight of any kind. Right now, my life is easy. I'm poor financially but rich in time.*

*I fear that if I change anything, get more goal-oriented, put myself out there, get back into the "game," I may have a manic episode, again, fry my brain, again, and end up in the hospital. I may not necessarily be able to recover as well as I have now. I feel that I have totally self-stigmatized myself into stability and don't see myself growing out of this disorder and getting back on the bandwagon.*

*It's both heartbreaking and a relief at the same time. Producing media is a hustle, and I'm no longer as sure of myself as I once was because I accept that I'm bipolar. Could you address the part of us that struggles with what we thought was real before our diagnosis and what should be a reality for us in the society and status quo in which we live, now that we're categorized as a stigmatized population here in the US?*

Clearly, this question was multi layered and deep, and I needed to ask Judy for clarification. So I asked:

*Are you saying that your bipolar disorder holds you back from hustling because you're afraid your career's intensity will push you into mania?*

Judy responded:

*Yes, exactly. I recognized, after being diagnosed, that much of what I'd accomplished to achieve the successes I'd had before*

*diagnosis was possible because I was unconsciously experiencing the symptoms of bipolar 1: racing ideas, grandiose thinking, sleeplessness/restlessness, having the expectation that others should know I'm a genius, planning for expansion of success before understanding the reality and hard work it takes to convince others you have talent and know what you're talking about, etc.*

*So, yes, I have a fear that I may have an episode if I go back to trying to pursue the life I lived before my diagnosis. How can I deal with this fear? Would it be better/smarter to move on and focus on the present moment and not try to push myself?*

This question addresses important points when it comes to managing ambitions. It also addresses a fear that's unique to people who live with an illness that changes their perception and makes them lose touch with reality.

One of the things Judy mentions, which I've seen other people grapple with, is the idea that mania allows you to do things you wouldn't otherwise be able to do because of the super energy and inflated outlook that lets you achieve all these things. Once you crash and burn, however, you're left thinking about what happened and the kind of person you became when you were on fire and rising to the top.

You may ask yourself: was that

really me, or was this just a manic-enhanced version of myself that should be avoided?

Severe mania can be destructive and disruptive: it can devastate people when they come down from its peak. There is often a huge mess to clean up consisting of things you did or neglected to do while you were manic. Additionally, if you become delusional, you can feel devastated that you lost control of your mind.

This can jolt your self-esteem, making you feel insecure. I've heard people say, "I didn't know I could think that way. How do I know I won't get like that again?" They can become afraid of doing anything that looks like it might put them on that merry-go-round again.

So that's the conflict Judy described. If she plays it safe by trying to keep from getting too close to this edge, she feels trapped in a stale existence that lacks fulfillment. On the flip side, she's stable now, and that's good. But she feels like she's living on autopilot.

Here are some thoughts about this.

First, it's helpful to recognize that you can't produce mania simply by being ambitious. You can have grand ambitions as part of your baseline personality.

Mania is an emotional state that increases your energy and impairs your judgment and impulse control. That's the state

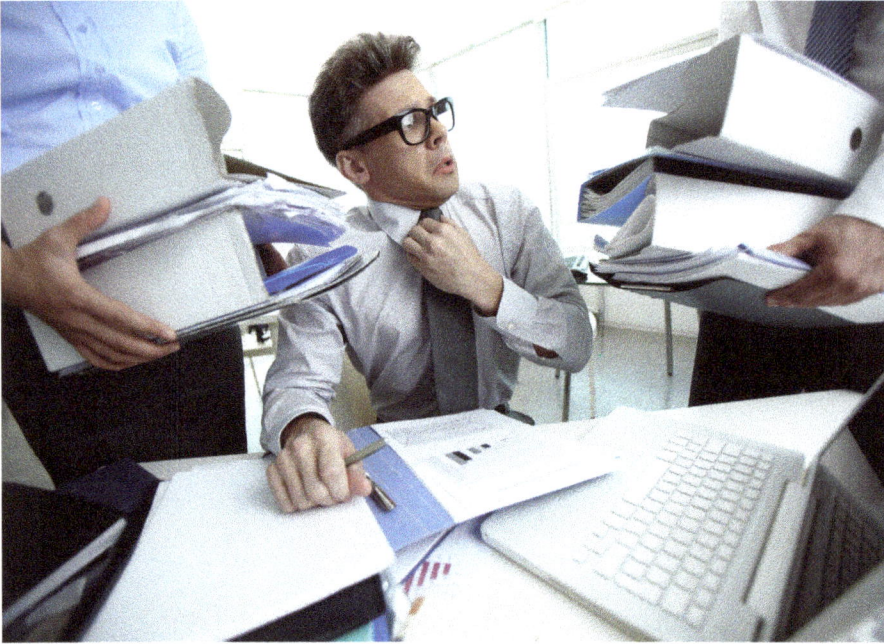

of mind that takes your baseline ambitions and grows them to grandiose and unrealistic levels.

Mania is part of bipolar disorder; it's not something that happens because you work really hard. So, in Judy's case, her first manifestation of the illness was probably mania. That mania fueled the hustle that helped build her business. She didn't get bipolar disorder because she was building a business. Some things she did to build the business may have been a byproduct of her mania. But she built her business over years. The mania probably crept in later in the process.

Since Judy desires to return to that business, I doubt that the business only prospered because she was manic. Usually, business ideas arising out of mania don't survive the mania's aftermath.

So, once you're back to your usual way of thinking, you realize that your ideas weren't realistic.

Sometimes it's hard to tell the difference between something you did because you were manic and something you would typically do, but the mania allowed you to do it faster, better, or more frequently.

As for returning to media work, bipolar disorder shouldn't mean that you can't pursue your interests. But it does mean you have to set limits on how much you work and prioritize self-care. With bipolar disorder, it's essential to stay on your treatment regimen and make sure you have good sleep hygiene.

These limitations may make it harder to do certain types of work. For example, it would not

be in your best interest to take a job that required you to be awake for 24–36 hours at a time regularly. Also, you wouldn't want to take a job where you couldn't take medication or see your doctor because you have to travel out of the country for six months at a time. These aren't absolute prohibitions. They're just examples of how your disorder creates limitations on the kind of work you do.

Now let's look at brain-frying issues resulting from working too hard. Usually, this surfaces when taking shortcuts to accomplish an objective or to do so faster. If you decelerate to accommodate self-care needs, the process may stunt your growth professionally. But slow growth is still growth, and that's important to keep in mind.

If your work is exciting, this doesn't mean you're manic or will become manic simply because you're excited. The over-the-top grandiose ideas come from the mania descending upon you and taking what you're already doing or thinking to another level.

Maintaining regularly scheduled doctor or therapy appointments and being aware of early signs that you're becoming manic are ways to avoid this. Knowing your early prodrome signs can help you, and then your doctor can make any necessary interventions to keep you from escalating into mania.

## CHAPTER 11

# Bipolar Disorder and Imposter Syndrome

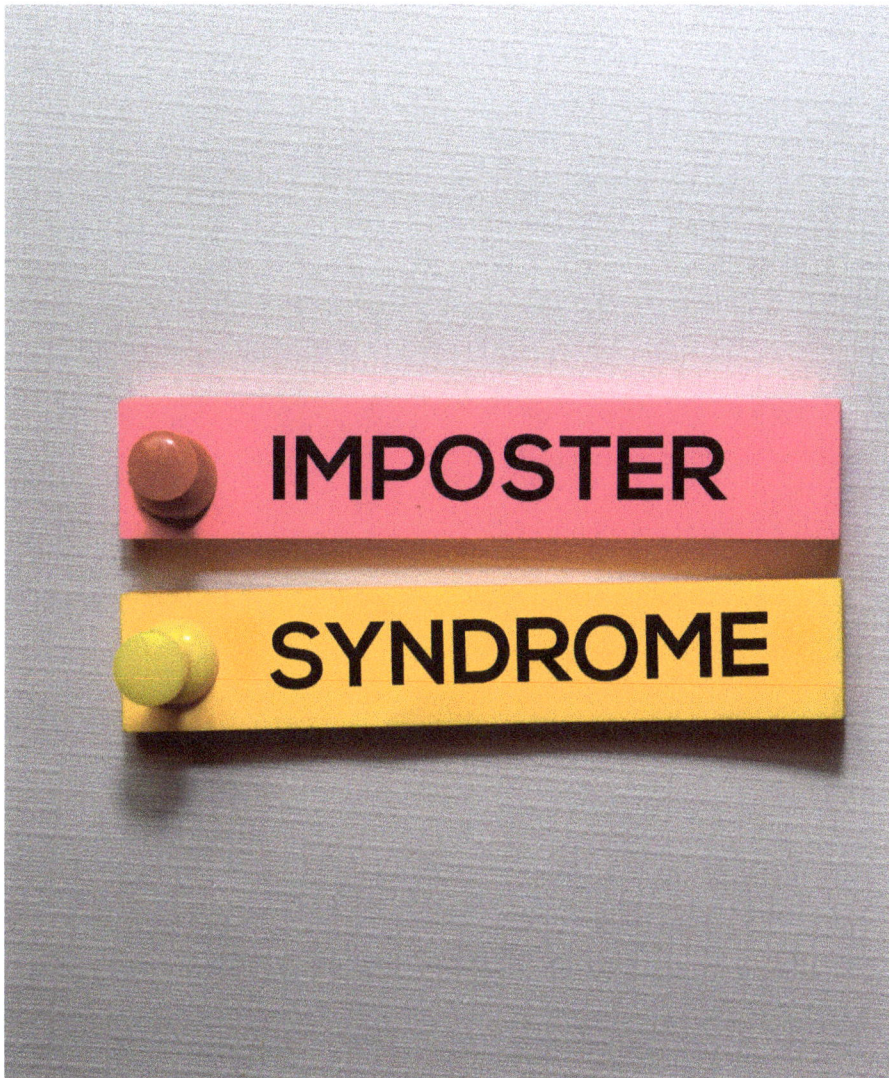

Here's the question.

*Sometimes a stable episode makes me feel like a fraud, or like maybe I'm just living a lie. So, what if I've wasted everyone's time, like my doctor fighting for me to get seen? It makes me feel guilty. But deep down, I know I'm not well. I keep a journal with all my episodes and such to hand to my psychiatrist, but, yeah, I just don't know. Sometimes this is more painful than my low episodes.*

There's not much written in the scientific literature about this imposter reaction, but it makes sense there wouldn't be much information, since people may be afraid to talk about this.

Do you ever feel like you've been faking your illness when you're well? This topic is based on a viewer question from my YouTube channel.

> YOU CAN FEEL LIKE AN IMPOSTER IF YOU DON'T INTERNALIZE THE ILLNESS. YOU BELIEVE IT DOESN'T BELONG TO THE "REAL" YOU.

Here's why this may happen.

## A DEFENSE MECHANISM

Real imposter syndrome happens when someone fails to internalize their accomplishments and skills and think they don't deserve their current position.

Likewise, with bipolar disorder, there can be a lack of internalization or taking ownership of the illness. This isn't simple denial—like saying to yourself, "There's nothing wrong with me." It's a deeper sense of "this isn't me." It's a defense mechanism you use to deal with the illness. And like imposter syndrome, you may feel at some level that you don't deserve all of the attention or help you get. Therefore (in your mind) you're a fraud for going through the motions as if you had something wrong with you.

If you're in between episodes, you can look back at your last episode and question your behavior. Here's what you might be thinking.

{ YOUR PSYCHOTIC THOUGHTS CAN FEEL SO UNRELATABLE THAT YOU CONCLUDE YOU MUST HAVE BEEN PRETENDING. }

How could I stay in bed for three days?

What normal person stares into space for 2 hours? I can't believe I did that. What's wrong with me?

These behaviors feel very foreign. They're removed from who you are at present. So what's the logical conclusion? You wonder whether maybe you made it all up? Even though you remember trading in your six-month-old car for a new Jaguar, now you begin to think that maybe you did that just to get attention or something like that. Because who does that? That's NOT you.

In this scenario, your behavior and thoughts while you were ill are so foreign in your mind that there's a significant disconnect when you try to match up who you believe you are with who that other person was. This complex thought interplay is known as ego-dystonic. The thoughts and behaviors don't match your current emotional state.

## DEPERSONALIZATION OR DEREALIZATION

Another thing that can contribute to this state is depersonalization and derealization. Derealization happens when you feel unreal and detached from your surroundings and environment. Your environment doesn't seem real. It's like being in a dream. Depersonalization is where you feel unreal and detached from your thoughts, your bodily sensations, and actions. It feels like you're observing yourself and your own thoughts.

You can experience derealization and depersonalization when you're manic or depressed. This can linger between episodes as well. Sometimes depersonalization can be extreme, but it can be more subtle, like feeling as if the past several months of symptoms weren't real. Believing you were faking your illness *can* be a way of saying, "I can't relate to the person I was when I was ill." To make sense of the episode, you may tell yourself that you were going through the motions and making up your symptoms. It's a conclusion you draw to piece together the disconnected story.

## YOU BECAME DELUSIONAL

Having psychotic episodes can also contribute to this feeling. This is an altered state during which you don't perceive things as they really are. When the psychosis resolves, you can't relate or connect to the thoughts you had. You can feel like you were playing a role or exaggerating things.

## WHAT CAN YOU DO ABOUT THIS?

You can keep a record of your episodes. You should note the timing of your symptoms and notice patterns of behavior. This helps you see an episode coming so you can take action to either prevent the episode or lessen its intensity.

## 5, 4, 3, 2, 1 EXERCISE

**5** Name 5 things you can see

**4** Name 4 things you can feel (real things, like the leather you're sitting on or the carpet under your feet)

**3** Name 3 things you can hear (like fingers tapping on a keyboard or the ticking of a clock)

**2** Name 2 things you can (or would like to) smell

**1** Name 1 good thing about yourself

Another reason to record your episodes is to remind yourself that you have an illness that comes and goes. When you're well, and have few to no symptoms, you can see what your illness looks like when you don't feel well.

Grounding exercises can also help. If you think what you're experiencing feels like depersonalization, you can employ grounding techniques. This will help you manage overwhelming feelings by reorienting you to the present. There are many ways to do this. One way is to wear a rubber band on your wrist. Snapping it helps to get you out of your head and bring you into the present. Another way is to do a sensory awareness exercise. It's called the 5, 4, 3, 2, 1 exercise. See the infographic.

## CHAPTER 12

# Can You Be Too Old To Get Bipolar Disorder?

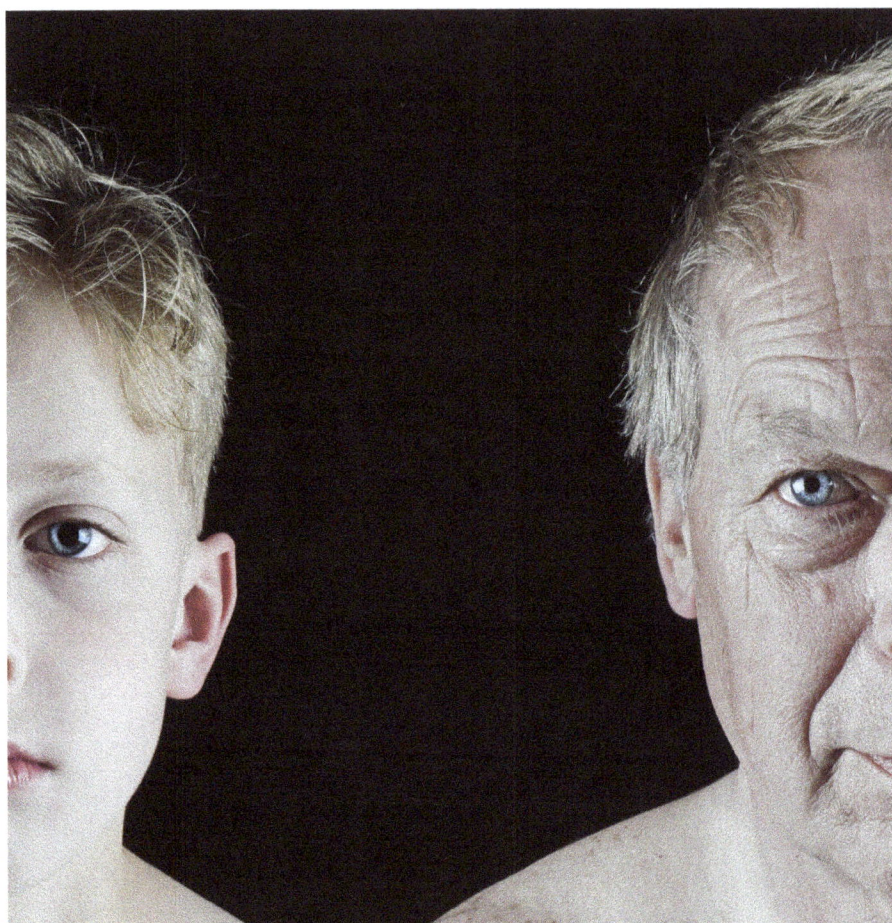

**B**ut there is a minority of people who develop bipolar disorder later, after the age of 40.

The International Society For Bipolar Disorders Task Force classified the illness into three categories. In this chapter, "manic" and "hypomanic" will be used interchangeably.

According to the task force classification, in early-onset bipolar disorder, the first manic episode occurs before the age of 40. Late-onset bipolar disorder is where the first manic episode occurs after the age of 50, and older age bipolar disorder is where the first manic episode occurs after the age of 60.

The typical age range in which people tend to develop bipolar disorder is 20 to 40. In Chapter 3, I talk about how the symptoms of bipolar disorder often show up as anxiety in the teenage years and progress to bipolar disorder in the early to late twenties.

ABOUT 25% OF PEOPLE HAVE THEIR FIRST MANIC EPISODE WHEN THEY ARE OVER 50.

dread. Thankfully, psychotic symptoms are less common and less severe with late-onset bipolar disorder than with early-onset. The psychosis (when untreated) combined with impulsivity and poor judgment can lead to destructive behavior during the episodes.

Because you are older and may have more medical issues, your doctor will have to pay close attention to how your medical conditions may affect you mentally. There tends to be more cognitive issues with late-onset bipolar disorder, like problems with memory, focus, and impaired problem-solving.

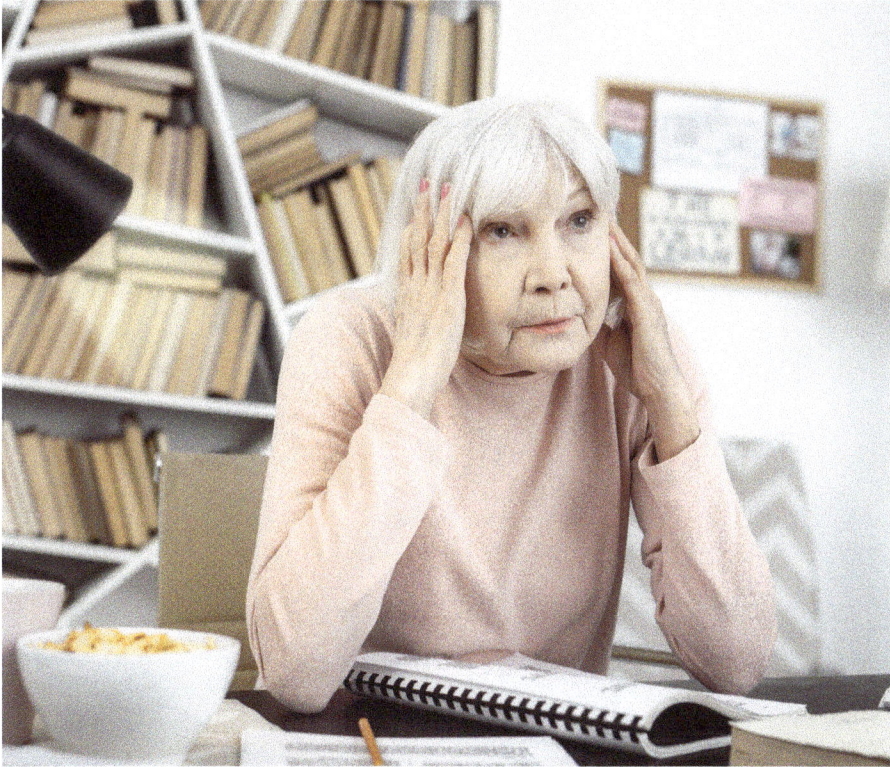

Notice that this criterion is based on when you have your first manic episode, and this is because mania is what distinguishes bipolar disorder from major depression. About 25% of people with bipolar disorder have an older age onset.

Let's say you have had three episodes of depression in the past fifteen years. How do you know whether you're going to develop bipolar disorder, and should your doctor prescribe a mood stabilizer now? The first answer is we don't have a way to reliably predict whether someone will develop mania at a later point. The second answer is that your doctor should not add a mood stabilizer to prevent you from having a manic episode if you are currently doing well on your antidepressant.

A soft sign that your depression may be bipolar depression is having symptoms of anxiety and agitation that don't respond to antidepressants. Some experts believe that depression with anxious distress is really a part of a bipolar spectrum illness. But we still haven't officially adopted that terminology.

One way we treat anxious depression is to add an antipsychotic or a mood stabilizer. That's not significantly different from the way we treat bipolar disorder, except with bipolar disorder, we try to eliminate the antidepressant so that you would only take mood stabilizers.

Sometimes it's hard to tell the difference between anxiety and mania. The differences are discussed in Chapter 24.

Having your depression become bipolar disorder doesn't have to be something you fear or

So, the take-away here is to be aware that if you have depression or have ever had recurring depressive episodes, there's still a possibility that you may have a late-onset episode of mania or hypomania. That doesn't mean you need to change anything now. It just means it's important to be aware that your doctor may need to treat you with different medications in future. Also, since we know that bipolar disorder responds well to having a structured schedule, you could try to maintain a regular schedule of eating and sleeping as a preventative measure.

Now is the time to improve your diet. A diet low in processed food reduces inflammation. Inflammatory markers are higher in people with depression and bipolar disorder. No one can predict the future, but you can do things to improve your outcome.

## CHAPTER 13

# What is considered to be a suicidal thought?

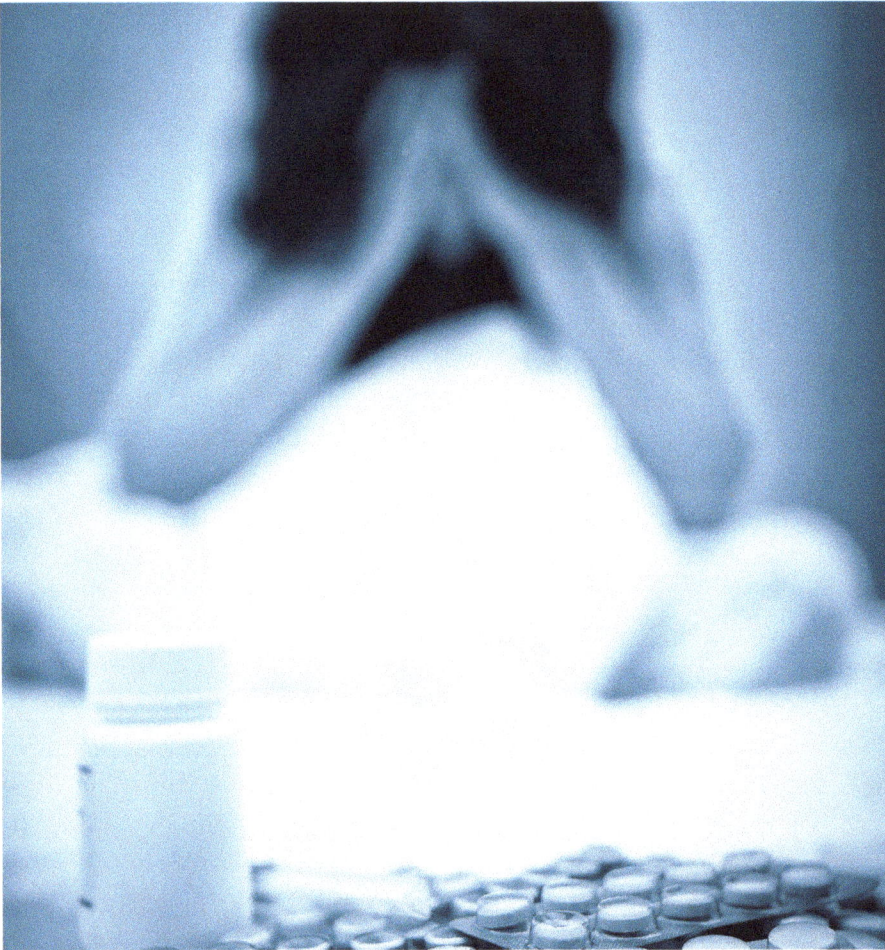

Here's the question.

*I'm wondering what are true suicidal thoughts? Is it being sure of your decision to where you're making plans without hesitation? Or can it also involve just having recurrent thoughts like, "I want to be over with this," "life isn't worth it," "I know how to do it, and, so, why don't I just do it?" I know my question may seem strange, but I'm starting to question myself and am conflicted and confused about this problem.*

We tend to characterize suicidal thoughts in two ways: active and passive. Active suicidal thinking is when you think through a plan. You may not actually make the plan, but you're thinking about options in your head. You may progress to executing the plan.

Another characteristic of suicidality is whether you have intention. You may have options you've thought of and even imagined carrying out. But because of your circumstances, such as having children or not

**Suicidality is a state of mind you can reach while either depressed or manic. A YouTube viewer asked how you know when you have a real suicidal thought.**

wanting to hurt the people around you, you say you'll never do it. Some people never have the intent because of their religious beliefs, even though they have the desire.

Passive suicidal thoughts are things like believing life isn't worth living or questioning the point of life. These are the kinds of thoughts mentioned in the question. These thoughts can stem from feeling hopeless and having the general sense you want the pain to end, or you want to free yourself from what seems like an impossible and unpleasant situation where you can see no light at the end of the tunnel. But you haven't thought through a plan concerning how to actively end your life. You might say something like, "If I were to walk out in front of a car and get hit, I wouldn't care." This is different from thinking about what street you should use if you had the nerve to actually do it.

Passive suicidal thoughts can become active, but many people never get to the point where they have active thoughts. They just ruminate passively in their head. Chronic passive thinking is still a problem and usually is a symptom of depression.

Also, some people just think of ending their lives as an option to keep open if the going gets too tough to handle. It's like having a fantasy escape plan. But they never seriously consider executing the plan. This kind of thinking doesn't necessarily mean you're depressed. Still,

it's dark thinking and can evolve into depression or active suicidal thinking.

There's another kind of thinking similar to suicidal thinking: an existential crisis. This thinking is focused on the meaning of your life. Does what you're doing in life have a purpose? Some can become distressed when thinking about their purpose and reason for existence. Thinking about this for long periods where there's no clear answer can lead to a sense of hopelessness, but it doesn't necessarily mean you're depressed.

On the other hand, this kind of thinking can signal early depression that's in development. It's commonly triggered by milestone events, such as graduating college and having to move back home because you can't find a job, getting divorced, or feeling stagnant in your career.

Self-harm can also be mistaken for suicidality. Sometimes ending your life is your intention, but people will often cut themselves to relieve tension or feel real. Some may take pill overdoses as a way to get help or to show others

that they're hurting.

If you're having suicidal thoughts, get help now. If you're under the care of a doctor or therapist, call them the first chance you get. If you don't have a doctor and you've been thinking about a plan, go to your nearest emergency room. Going to an emergency room doesn't mean you'll be admitted to the hospital. But they'll assess you and make referrals for help outside of a hospital when they believe you're safe to leave. If you don't have a doctor or can't get to a hospital, call a suicide prevention hotline for support and help. The National Suicide Prevention Lifeline is one such resource that provides 24-hour access for support. Their phone number is 800-273-8255.

Another thing you can do is develop a suicide safety plan. This is something that's best done with the help of a doctor or therapist. But if you don't have one, you can still think through these exercises yourself. The safety plan is a list of coping strategies and support sources to use when feeling suicidal. Here's a six-step safety plan based on the Stanley 2011 study referenced in the Bibliography. Write down these steps.

## STEP 1: IDENTIFY WARNING SIGNS

Ask yourself: what's going on when you become suicidal? Think about your behaviors and thought processes. An example of where someone's transitioning from

> AN EXISTENTIAL CRISIS CAN MAKE YOU FEEL HOPELESS, BUT IT DOESN'T MEAN YOU'RE DEPRESSED.

passive to active suicidal thinking would be thinking about buying a gun and researching places where one can be purchased. An example behavior may consist of pushing people away and isolating yourself.

## STEP 2: WRITE DOWN COPING STRATEGIES

These are things you can do on your own to help you not act on suicidal thoughts. Examples of this might be to go for a walk outside or watch a movie to help take your mind off things. It doesn't need to be something that sounds healthy, like going on a run. It should be something that you can do easily, that gives you pleasure.

If this doesn't work, go to step 3.

## STEP 3: IDENTIFY SOCIAL CONTACTS OR SETTINGS THAT DISTRACT YOU FROM THE CRISIS

Ask yourself:

- Who do you like to be around when you want to get your mind off things?
- Is there a place you can go that makes you feel good?

If you choose to go out with a friend, it's okay if they're a casual friend. This isn't a step where you tell the person what's going on. You're keeping it light. You want the situation itself to distract you. An example of step 3 might consist of sitting in a coffee shop or bookstore and watching people.

If this doesn't help enough, then move to step 4.

## STEP 4: ENGAGE FRIENDS OR FAMILY MEMBERS

In this step, list three or more people in order of priority, with the first person on the list being the most supportive of you. This would be someone in whom you can freely confide about your crisis. This is your network of supportive friends and family members.

If this doesn't work, go to step 5.

## STEP 5: CONTACT A PROFESSIONAL

Create a list of your providers, local urgent care centers, or hotlines. The list should include the phone numbers of these providers.

## STEP 6: MAKE YOUR ENVIRONMENT SAFE

Eliminate things like guns or large bottles of pills. If you get a 90-day supply of medications, take out only enough for a week at a time and put them in a pill organizer. Then give the rest to a trusted friend or family member. Even though this is the last step, include it as part of your plan, even if the earlier steps helped.

The last question to ask yourself is this: **What's one person or thing currently in my life that is important enough for me to stay alive?** Write this one thing down on your list so you can keep yourself focused on the big reason

you will implement the six-step safety plan.

Remember that most suicide attempts are impulsive. You convince yourself your situation will improve if everything's over—for good. You also convince yourself that people won't care if you do this—so it's not hurting anyone. But that is distorted, in-the-moment thinking. The reality you don't appreciate is that the collateral damage from suicide runs deep and wide. It's like a nuclear blast leaving permanent pain behind.

Use this template to help you write out a plan. Make a copy for yourself and give a copy to close friends and family members. Give a copy also to your therapist. If you prefer to keep things on your phone, there's an app called MY3 with a safety plan. It even allows you to email it to people.

You may reprint this template and the worksheets in Chapter 19 by downloading them here: https://markspsychiatry.com/handbook-sheets

> MOST SUICIDE ATTEMPTS ARE IMPULSIVE. YOU CONVINCE YOURSELF THAT IT'S THE RIGHT THING TO DO AT THE MOMENT.

# MY SAFETY PLAN

**STEP 1**
### IDENTIFY WARNING SIGNS
What are your thoughts and behaviors?

**STEP 2**
### IDENTIFY COPING STRATEGIES
What can you do to soothe yourself?

**STEP 3**
### IDENTIFY SOCIAL DISTRACTIONS
List people and places

**STEP 4**
### LIST FAMILY AND CLOSE FRIENDS
You can tell them your true feelings

**STEP 5**
### LIST DOCTOR, THERAPIST OR AGENCY
List the name and phone number

**STEP 6**
### MAKE YOUR ENVIRONMENT SAFE
Remove all things you can use for harm

**WHAT IS ONE PERSON OR THING THAT IS IMPORTANT ENOUGH FOR YOU TO WANT TO STAY ALIVE?**

## CHAPTER 14

# What is Classic Bipolar vs. Atypical?

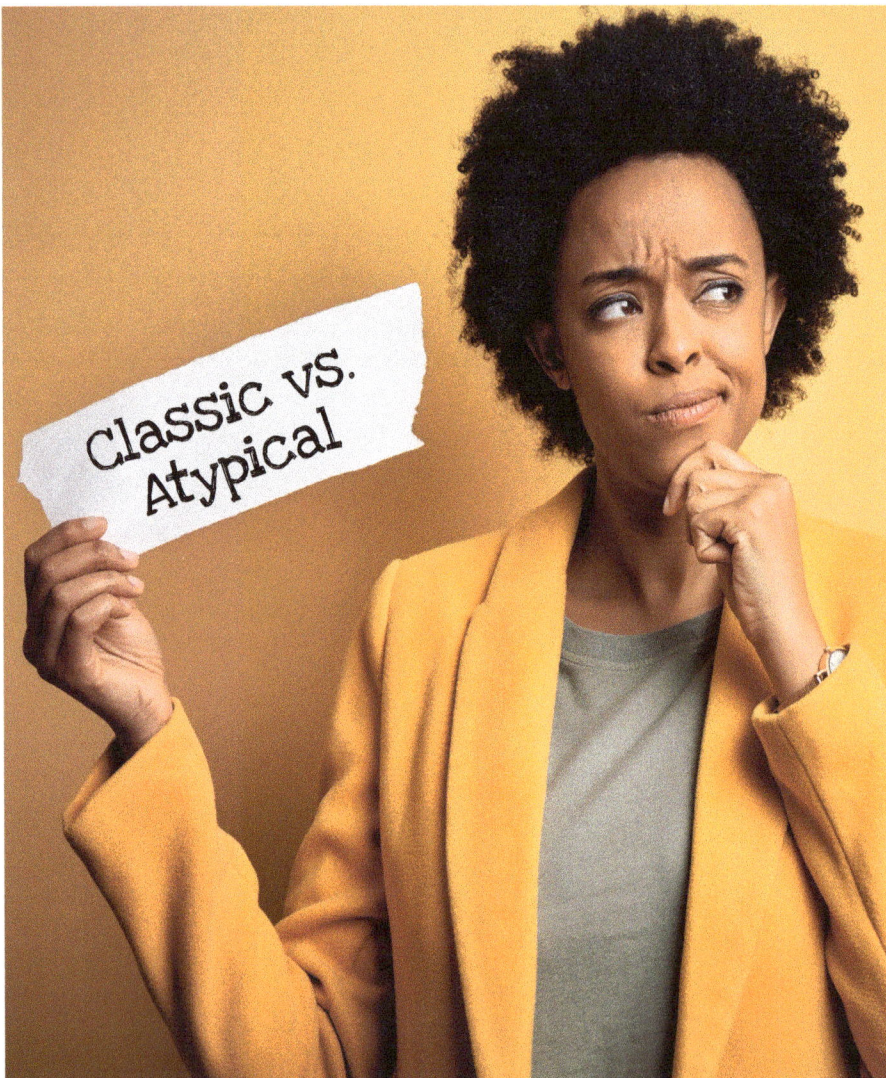

**T**hese have been referred to as a classic or textbook pattern and an atypical pattern. These aren't official subtypes of bipolar disorder in the diagnostic manual. Instead, this is a clinical description of two ways bipolar disorder can manifest.

This distinction is important because the classic form of bipolar disorder tends to respond better to lithium. The atypical form tends to respond better to anticonvulsant mood stabilizers, like valproic acid and lamotrigine, and atypical antipsychotic medications, like aripiprazole and quetiapine.

I use and define a lot of terms in this chapter. Understanding clinical terms will help you in any discussion about them. Sometimes your doctor can slip

In defining bipolar disorder, we've talked about the two types: 1 and 2. Within these two types, there are two ways the disorder looks and behaves.

> **CLASSIC BIPOLAR DISORDER TENDS TO RESPOND BETTER TO LITHIUM.**

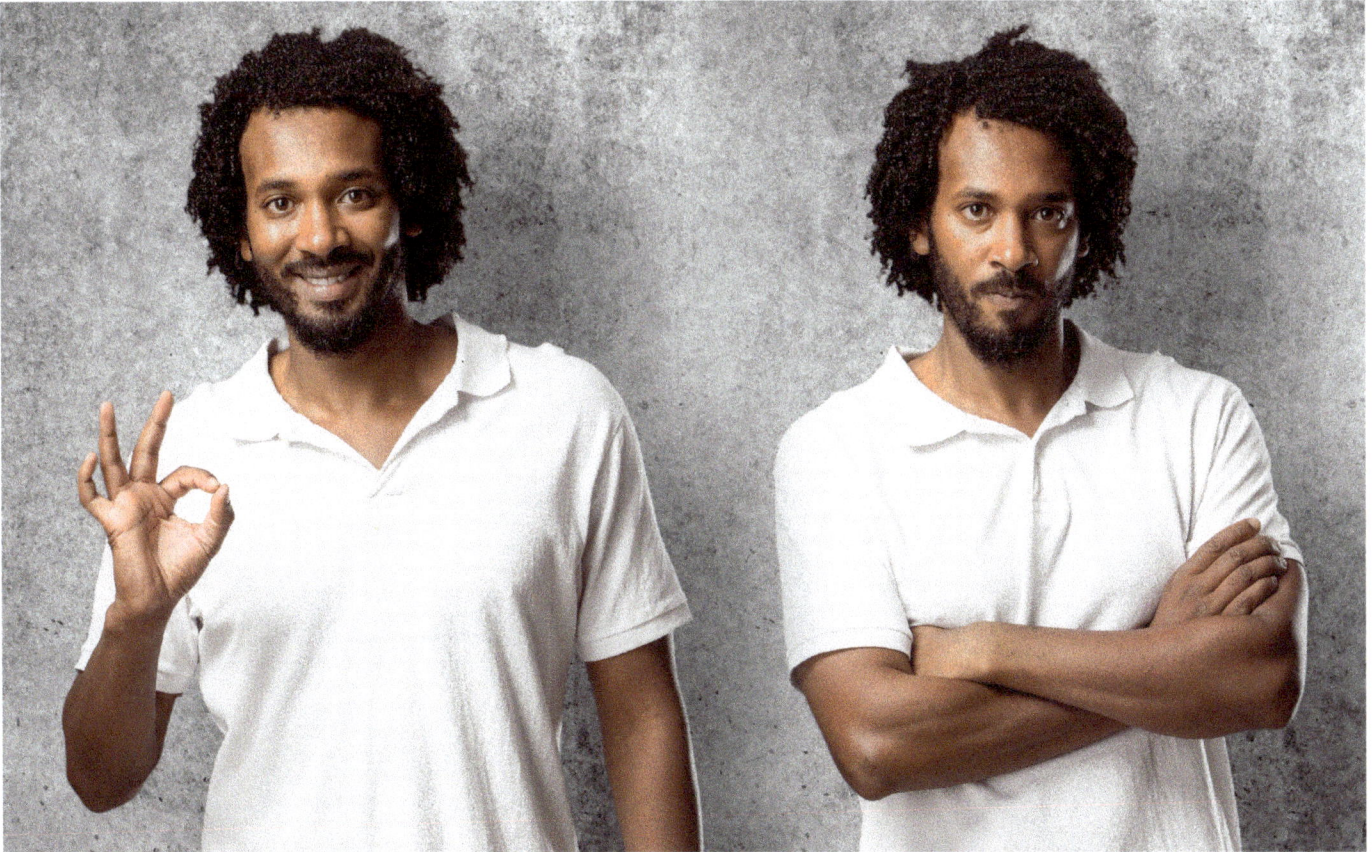

and use these terms without thinking about it.

## ATYPICAL ANTIPSYCHOTICS

They're called atypical because they block dopamine *and* serotonin, whereas the older antipsychotics, like haloperidol, block only dopamine. The first generation of antipsychotics focused only on treating psychosis. Then, in 1990, the first of the second generation of antipsychotic medications started with clozapine. These are the antipsychotics mostly used today, especially in treating bipolar disorder and treatment-resistant depression.

Here's a comparison of classic bipolar and atypical bipolar disorder.

For hypomania and mania, you'll start with euphoric or happy/grandiose mania with classic bipolar disorder. As you get older, your manias generally become more irritable.

With atypical, you'll get predominately dysphoria or dark moods. You can also get mixed states.

With classic bipolar, you'll have a full recovery between episodes and you can have long periods in between episodes. When you're not having an episode, you're back to your baseline state, and that can last for months or years before another episode.

With atypical, you tend to have leftover symptoms of lesser intensity in between episodes. It may not feel like you fully

recovered from your last depression. The clinical term for the leftover symptoms is subsyndromal. They're symptoms that, standing alone, aren't severe enough to be diagnosed as an illness or syndrome. But, here, they're remnant symptoms of your bipolar illness.

Rapid cycling means having more than four episodes in a year. It is more common with atypical bipolar and rare with the classic form. You don't tend to have other disorders like anxiety, addictions, or obsessive-compulsive disorder (OCD) with the classic form. These other illnesses are called comorbidities because they co-occur with other illnesses.

"Morbidity" or "morbid" is a clinical term for a disease state. If you ever read or hear someone

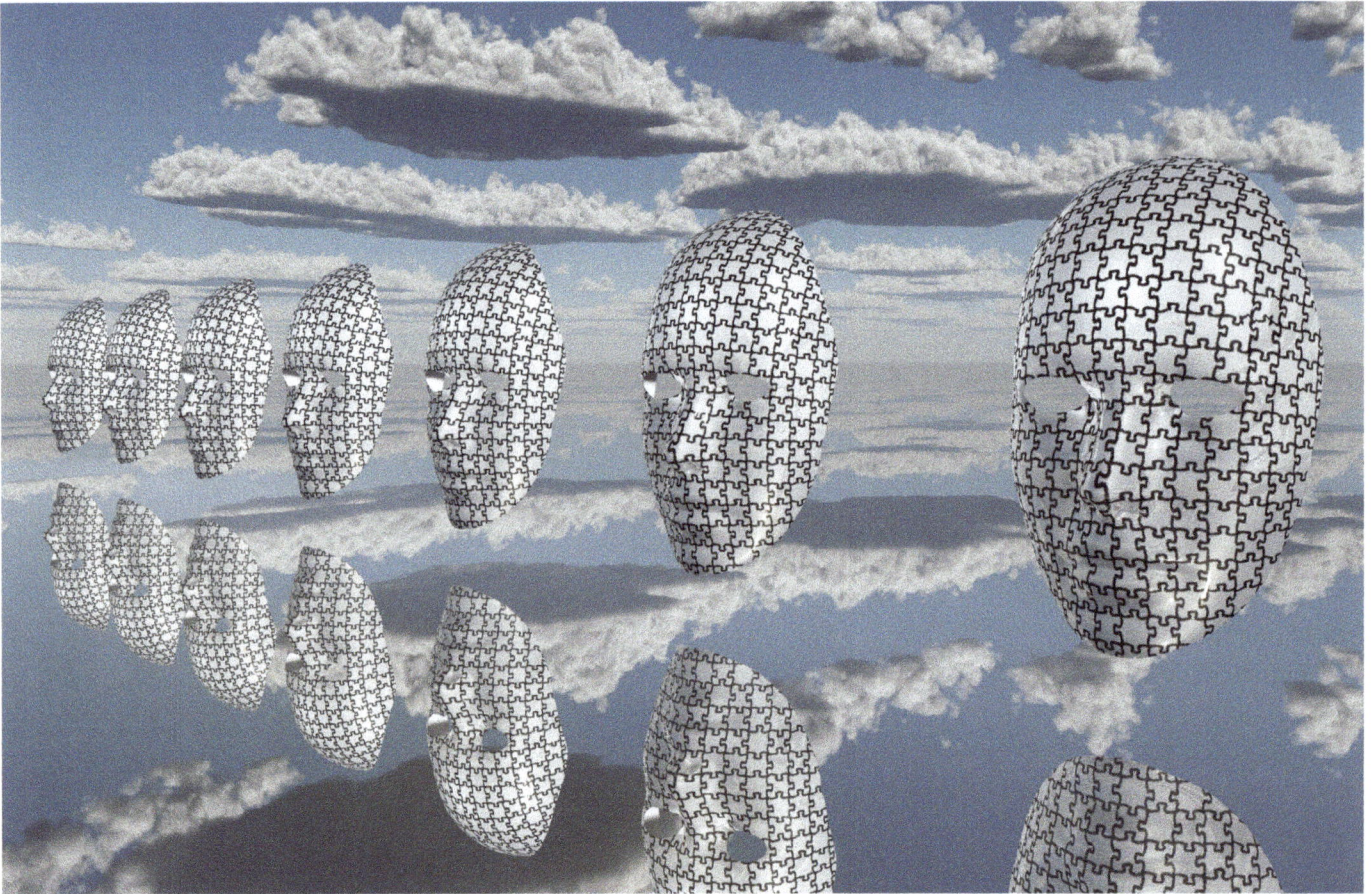

refer to your pre-morbid state, it refers to how you were before you were ill. And if you have several illnesses, such as ADHD, anxiety, bipolar disorder, etc., they're considered comorbidities.

So, we tend to think of classic bipolar as being purer and not affected by other illnesses.

{ PEOPLE WITH CLASSIC BIPOLAR TEND TO HAVE HIGH ENERGY AND BE NATURAL LEADERS. }

The age of onset of classic bipolar disorder tends to be about 15–19, and for atypical, it's earlier, like 10–15. These are average ages when you start showing symptoms that can later be diagnosed as bipolar disorder. Generally, psychiatric illnesses that take shape in a defined way in childhood tend to evolve into a more severe form in adulthood. It's as if the illness has more time to gain momentum and become a stronger version of itself.

As for personality style, with classic bipolar disorder, people tend to either have a "normal" personality that doesn't cause problems, or they have what's called a hyperthymic personality. Hyperthymic is a term describing someone who's naturally "high

energy," or "a people person" who tends to be a leader.

With atypical bipolar disorder, you see more personality disorders like borderline personality or cyclothymic temperament. Cyclothymic temperament is a psychological construct, not a diagnosis.  A construct is a concept or theory that someone has developed. Your temperament refers to the hardwiring with which you were born. If you have a cyclothymic temperament, you're essentially hardwired to be moodier and emotionally reactive. This reactivity comes from being more sensitive in your interactions with others.

The last comparison concerns genetics. With classic bipolar

disorder, there is often a history of someone in your family having it because this disorder is strongly heritable. Heritable means capable of being inherited or passed down to another generation.

In psychiatry, the two most heritable disorders are bipolar disorder and schizophrenia. If you have a first-degree relative with this illness, it's not a given you'll get it, too, but your odds of developing it are greater than those of someone who has no family history of this condition. A first-degree relative would be someone who shares half your DNA, like a parent or sibling. A cousin or uncle would be a second-degree relative.

Classic bipolar is more common than bipolar disorder and runs in families. With atypical bipolar disorder, the family history of it is usually murkier. You may have relatives who have other disorders like depression, schizophrenia, or other illnesses. In general, psychiatric illness can run in families such that you can have an uncle with schizophrenia while you end up having depression. You didn't inherit the same illness as your uncle, but you still have an other type of mental disorder.

The classic bipolar picture is actually less common than the atypical presentation. The word "atypical" makes it sound as if it's not the usual. It's called atypical because when Emil Kraepelin first discussed bipolar disorder, it was the classic form which he first defined. Later, this other variation became recognized. So, it's similar to the antipsychotic story. The newer, second-generation antipsychotics are called atypicals because they're essentially a spin-off of the older ones. But they're more commonly used now than the typical ones.

The primary significance of recognizing these differences is that classic bipolar tends to be more responsive to lithium, which has many benefits, including being neuroprotective. This means it protects nerve cells in your brain from injury or degeneration. Even though lithium can sometimes make people feel cognitively slowed or dulled, it's been shown to slow the onset and progression of dementia. But it's not always an easy drug to take, and it has significant side effects.

Still, if you have a more atypical presentation of your bipolar disorder, you'll probably get better results with anticonvulsants and atypical antipsychotic medications.

The next section addresses medication options.

# TREATMENT OPTIONS

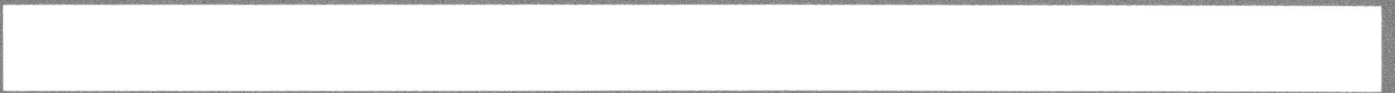

_____

## CHAPTER 15

# How Lithium Is Used To Treat Bipolar Disorder

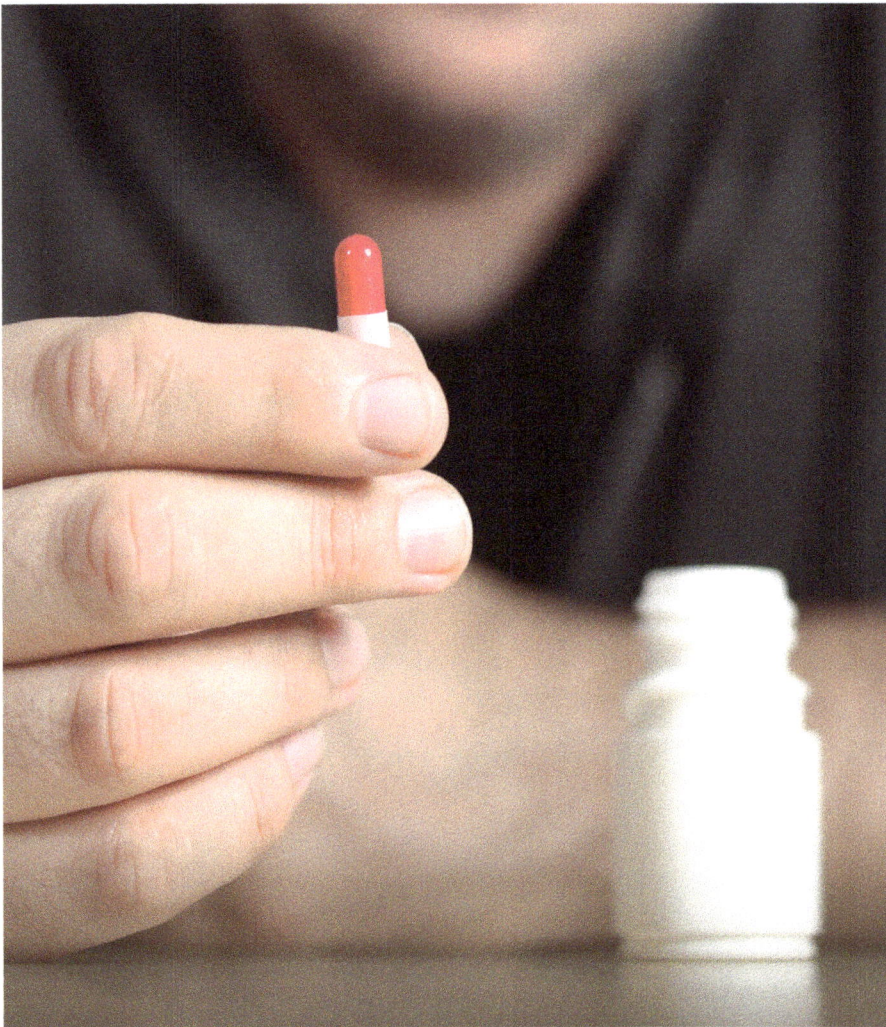

In the case of mixed features, the recommended first choice is an antipsychotic medication like quetiapine. We use second-generation antipsychotic medications as mood stabilizers in bipolar disorder.

One thing lithium does better than other medications is reduce suicidal thinking. The only other medication addressing this at the same level is ketamine, which is commonly used to treat resistant unipolar depression.

Lithium has neuroprotective effects such as increasing brain-derived neurotrophic factor and reducing nerve cell death (called apoptosis). It also reduces oxidative stress that results from multiple episodes of mania and depression.

Lithium is the first recommended treatment for bipolar disorder, especially when you have classic bipolar disorder. Lithium is not a good choice when you have mixed episodes or rapid cycling.

DESPITE ITS MANY SIDE EFFECTS, LITHIUM HAS POSITIVE EFFECTS ON THE BRAIN.

These are just some of lithium's benefits. Still, lithium has significant potential side effects. Some are short-term and resolve after discontinuing the medication, while others are long-term and, in some cases, permanent.

## LITHIUM SIDE EFFECTS

Lithium can cause weight gain, tiredness, and fuzzy thinking, similar to side effects resulting from other mood stabilizers. But lithium also has side effects that develop from long-term use. The first long-term side effect is it can cause your thyroid to produce inadequate amounts of thyroid hormone. Some people who take lithium on a long-term basis need thyroid supplementation. Some will stop taking lithium because of this problem, even though nothing else works as well.

The second long-term side effect involves your kidneys.  A decline in kidney function naturally happens as you get older. But long-term lithium use can accelerate this process, and you can develop diabetes insipidus. This is different from diabetes mellitus, where you get elevated blood sugar levels. With insipidus, your kidneys don't adequately concentrate your urine. You need to urinate frequently and suffer from excessive thirst.

Diabetes insipidus can happen even within the first few weeks of taking lithium. It usually resolves on its own but can persist in about 25% of people.

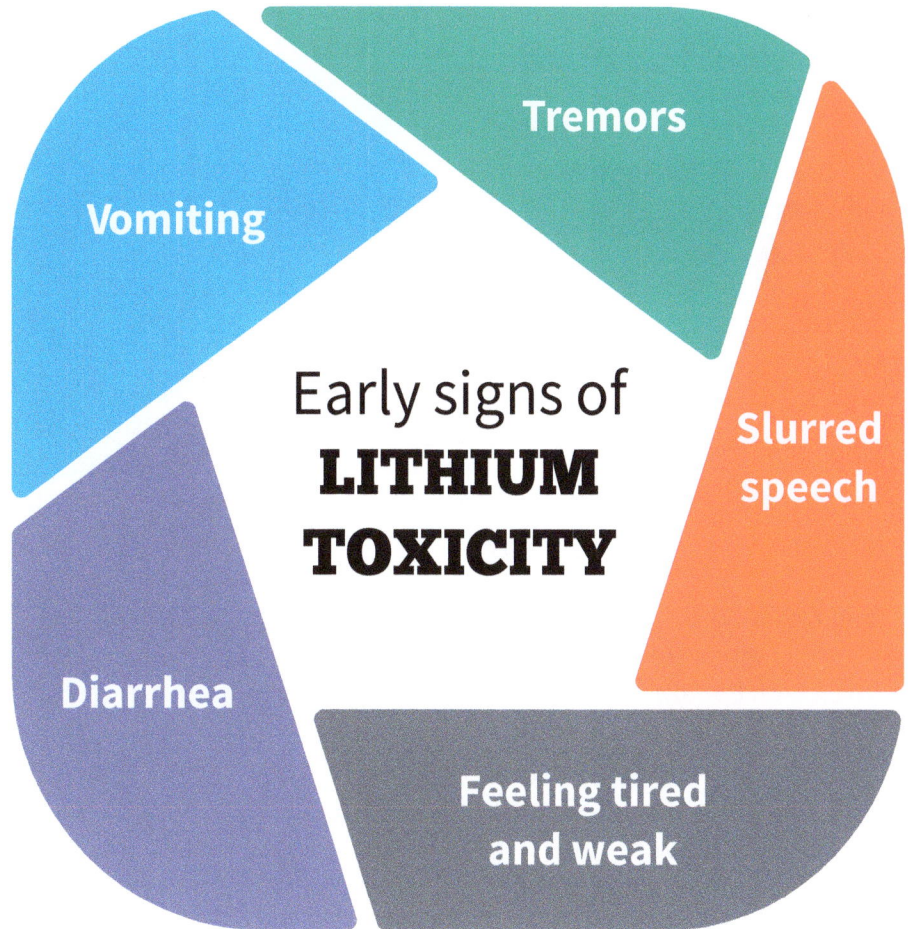

Early signs of
# LITHIUM TOXICITY

- Tremors
- Vomiting
- Slurred speech
- Diarrhea
- Feeling tired and weak

Sometimes this problem can be helped by taking the full dose of lithium at bedtime. If the problem doesn't resolve, you'll likely need to switch to a different mood stabilizer. If detected early, diabetes insipidus is often reversible within weeks.

Lithium can negatively affect kidneys when it becomes too concentrated and reaches toxic levels in your blood. So, it's important to have your lithium levels checked regularly. Also, it's important to stay hydrated. If you lose a lot of fluid from excessive sweating, diarrhea, or vomiting, watch for signs of lithium toxicity.

Early signs of lithium toxicity include the following:

- Tremors
- Slurred speech
- Feeling tired and weak
- Diarrhea
- Vomiting.

Diarrhea and vomiting can cause lithium toxicity because of resulting fluid loss, but they can also occur if you become toxic. If you notice any of these symptoms, you should go to an emergency room or urgent care to be evaluated.

Inform your doctors if you're on lithium so they can check

for any drug interactions from medications already prescribed. If you have pain problems, watch your consumption of non steroidal anti-inflammatory medications like ibuprofen or naproxen. This class of medication can increase lithium levels.

## WHAT ABOUT LITHIUM OROTATE?

This is a version of over-the-counter lithium that has a lower dose than prescription lithium. Lithium orotate delivers about 1/5 of the amount of lithium you get with lithium carbonate. Some studies have shown mental health benefits to people living in communities where lithium is added to drinking water (Kapusta 2015).

A downside to taking over-the-counter lithium is not having clear guidelines concerning what's effective. Also, you have to monitor yourself when it comes to becoming dehydrated or keep up with other medications that could raise your level. How much the micro-dosing affects your thyroid or kidneys is still unclear.

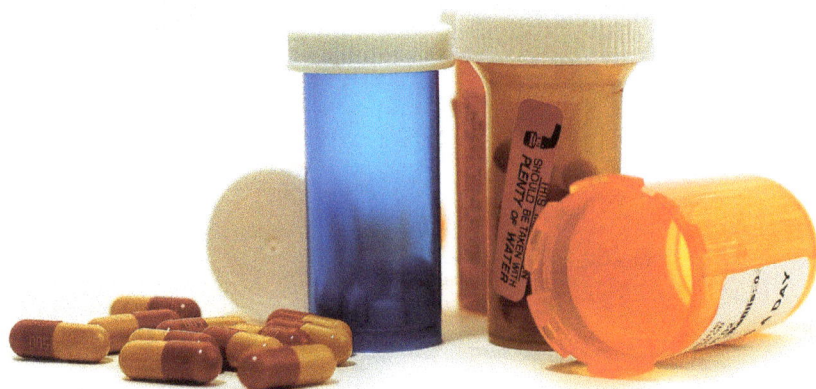

Prescription lithium comes with significant potential side effects. Still, it's an effective treatment for bipolar disorder, though it isn't guaranteed to work. You may experience mixed symptoms when taking it or, for whatever reason, you just don't feel comfortable with this medication. In that case, there are other medication options for you and your doctor to consider.

## CHAPTER 16

# The Right Mood Stabilizers For the Right Phase

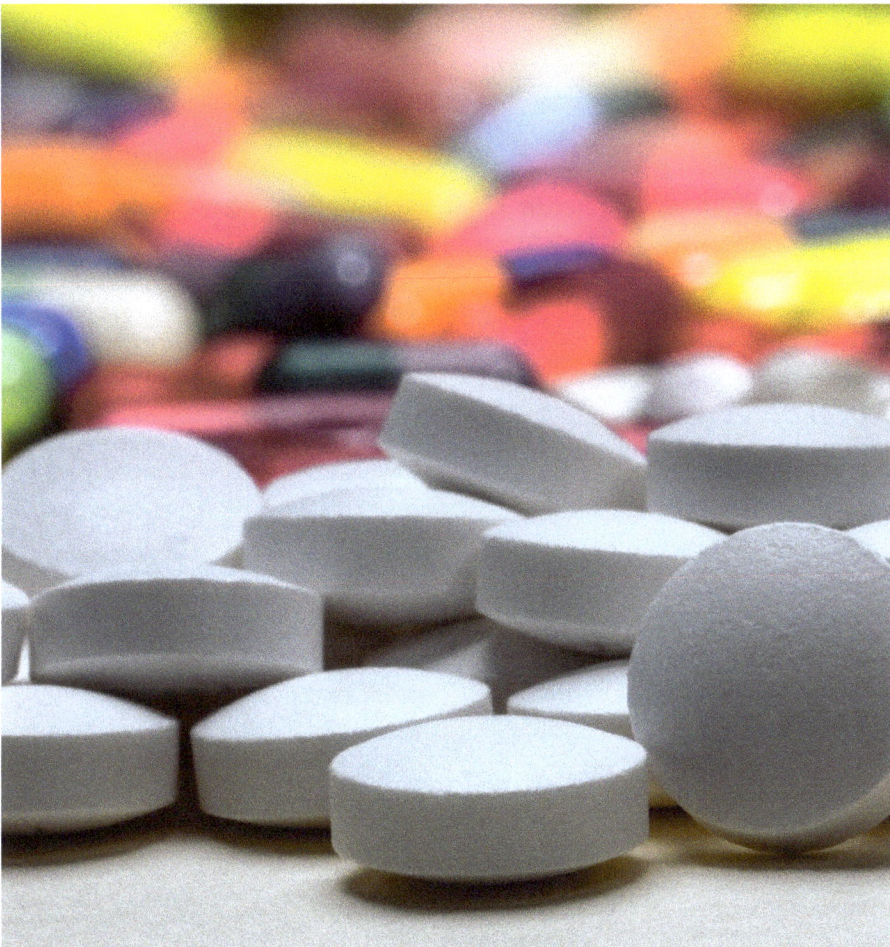

**A**nticonvulsant medications are called anticonvulsants because they treat seizures. Neurologists use them for seizure management, but they can also be prescribed to treat migraine headaches. Psychiatrists mainly use them to treat bipolar disorder. They also have off-label uses to treat other conditions, such as anxiety.

The antipsychotic medications commonly used are second-generation atypical antipsychotics. They work robustly for mood stabilization even if you do not have any psychotic symptoms.

Aside from lithium, the primary medications used to treat bipolar disorder are mood stabilizers, which fall into two categories: anticonvulsants and antipsychotics.

ANTIDEPRESSANTS, AREN'T GENERALLY USED TO TREAT BIPOLAR DISORDER BECAUSE THEY OFTEN TRIGGER RAPID CYCLING OF EPISODES.

Off-label prescription use refers to prescribing a drug to treat a condition for which the drug is not approved to treat. When medications are developed, they are approved by the US Food and Drug Administration (FDA) for specific problems or conditions (called indications). These indications are included on the medication's label. The label is more than the sticker affixed to the outside of the bottle from the pharmacy. It's the printed information about the drug that includes the generic medication name, approved indications, warnings, dosages, drug interactions, and other details required by the FDA for disclosure. The label is usually a few pages long and sometimes will come attached to your pill bottle or box.

Once the medication is being widely used, doctors and researchers may find that the medication helps another condition. If the company that developed the drug does not undergo the expensive process of getting FDA approval for another indication, it may become accepted practice among doctors to use the medication for the off-label condition.

Antidepressants, generally, aren't used to treat bipolar disorder because they often trigger rapid cycling of episodes. The Systematic Treatment Enhancement Program–Bipolar Disorder (STEP-BD) is a federally funded long-term study designed to see what treatments work best for treating bipolar disorder. It is an authoritative study upon which medical professionals rely for treatment recommendations. The study showed that people with bipolar disorder taking antidepressants experienced many more depressive episodes.

Often you will need to take a combination of medications because each medication is designed to treat different aspects of the disorder. The main four phases targeted in treating bipolar disorder are acute depression, acute mania, mixed states, and the maintenance phase.

Acute refers to the active state you're in and is relatively recent. The maintenance phase is the period in between episodes when things have stabilized.

Not all of the medications work for every phase. You could be prescribed a medication to treat mania and, once it resolves, become depressed. Then the original medication for the mania won't improve your depression.

These are the FDA-approved medications for acute mania.

The antipsychotic medications are: aripiprazole (Abilify®), asenapine (Saphris®), cariprazine (Vraylar®), olanzapine (Zyprexa®), quetiapine (Seroquel®), risperidone (Risperdal®), and ziprasidone (Geodon®).

The anticonvulsants are: carbamazepine, lithium, and valproic acid.

All three of these anticonvulsant medications require blood level testing. So, if you take them, you'll need to have your blood level checked frequently. Achieving a range-appropriate level may take several weeks or months, after which your doctor may check your levels for monitoring purposes one to two times a year.

For bipolar depression, the only medications approved to treat this phase are cariprazine (Vraylar®), lurasidone (Latuda®), quetiapine (Seroquel®), and Symbyax® (which is a combination pill that includes olanzapine and fluoxetine). Notice there are no anticonvulsants on this list.

For mixed episodes, the approved medications are aripiprazole (Abilify®), asenapine (Saphris®), cariprazine (Vraylar®), olanzapine (Zyprexa®), quetiapine (Seroquel®), risperidone (Risperdal®), and ziprasidone (Geodon®). There are no anticonvulsants on this list.

The maintenance phase is when you're out of your depression or mania. You may have some residual symptoms, but you don't have intense symptoms that cause significant dysfunction in your life. You may still have some symptoms, but they will be significantly

COMBINATION THERAPY IS COMMONLY USED TO TREAT BIPOLAR DISORDER BECAUSE DIFFERENT MEDICATIONS HAVE DIFFERENT PURPOSES.

# Bipolar Medication Indications
## What They Are Supposed To Treat

| BIPOLAR MANIA | BIPOLAR DEPRESSION | BIPOLAR MIXED | BIPOLAR MAINTENANCE |
|---|---|---|---|
| Abilify (aripiprazole)<br>**Saphris** (asenapine)<br>**Vraylar** (cariprazine)<br>Zyprexa (olanzapine)<br>Seroquel (quetiapine)<br>Risperdal (risperidone)<br>Geodon (ziprasidone)<br>Lithium*<br>Tegretol (carbamaze-pine)*<br>Depakote (valproic acid)* | Vraylar (cariprazine)<br><br>Seroquel (quetiapine)<br><br><br><br><br><br>**Latuda** (lurasidone)<br>Symbyax (olanzapine/fluoxetine) | Abilify (aripiprazole)<br>**Saphris** (asenapine)<br>**Vraylar** (cariprazine)<br>Zyprexa (olanzapine)<br>Seroquel (quetiapine)<br>Risperdal (risperidone)<br>Geodon (ziprasidone) | Abilify (aripiprazole)<br>**Saphris** (asenapine)<br><br>Zyprexa (olanzapine)<br>Seroquel (quetiapine)<br><br>Geodon (ziprasidone)<br>Lithium*<br><br>Lamictal (lamotrigine)* |

Medications in bold are brand names only; all the rest have a generic equivalent (generic name in parenthesis)

*Lithium, Tegretol, Depakote and Lamictal are the non-antipsychotic mood stabilizers*

| Weight Gain | | | | | Sedation | | |
|---|---|---|---|---|---|---|---|
| **Worst** | **Moderate** | **Lower** | **Least** | | **Worst** | **Moderate** | **Least** |
| olanzapine (10–30 pounds average) | quetiapine<br>risperidone<br>cariprazine | asenapine | aripiprazole<br>lurasidone<br>ziprasidone | | olanzapine<br>quetiapine | asenapine<br>cariprazine<br>lurasidone<br>risperidone<br>ziprasidone | aripiprazole |

improved and much more manageable.

Maintenance medications work best to extend the length of time between episodes, prevent them from occurring, or decrease a returning episode's intensity. These medicines are like having armed guards protecting your perimeter to keep the enemy from penetrating the barrier.

Antipsychotic medications approved for the maintenance phase are aripiprazole (Abilify®), asenapine (Saphris®), quetiapine (Seroquel®), ziprasidone (Geodon®), and olanzapine (Zyprexa®).

The anticonvulsants are: lamotrigine (Lamictal®) and lithium.

Being FDA-approved signifies that these drugs have been shown to be beneficial for a specific phase of the illness. Your doctor can still prescribe medications that aren't approved for a specific phrase, but they may not work as well because they lack the track record of success in treating that phase. Still, the medication may be effective for you.

Combination therapy is commonly used to treat bipolar disorder because different medications have different purposes. Medication that helps get you better may

not be effective at keeping you well. Treatment for bipolar disorder often requires changing medications because of side effect tolerance. For example, quetiapine is recommended to treat all four phases. But it's also sedating and causes more weight gain than some of the other medications.

Lamotrigine isn't as effective as quetiapine, but its side effects are better tolerated. So, adding quetiapine to treat an acute manic or depressive episode is a strategy your doctor may employ. Then your doctor could simultaneously add lamotrigine as the drug you remain on after the episode has passed.

# EXAMPLE MEDICATION STRATEGY
## ACUTE MANIA OR DEPRESSION

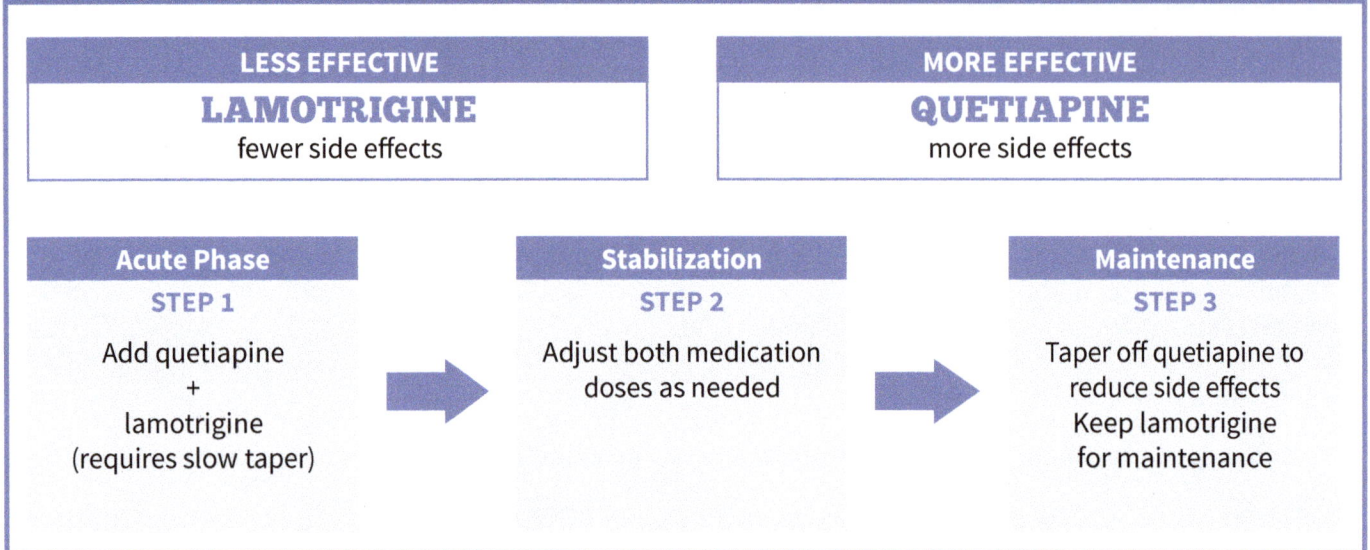

| LESS EFFECTIVE | MORE EFFECTIVE |
| --- | --- |
| **LAMOTRIGINE** fewer side effects | **QUETIAPINE** more side effects |

| Acute Phase | Stabilization | Maintenance |
| --- | --- | --- |
| STEP 1 | STEP 2 | STEP 3 |
| Add quetiapine + lamotrigine (requires slow taper) | Adjust both medication doses as needed | Taper off quetiapine to reduce side effects Keep lamotrigine for maintenance |

Quetiapine will do the heavy lifting when it comes to treating the mania or depression. Once the episode has resolved, your doctor can taper you off the quetiapine to reduce side effects and keep you on lamotrigine for maintenance.

This is just one example of a possible combination therapy addressing different phases of the illness. Sometimes you may need to stay on two medications to remain stable.

That's the reasoning behind combining certain medications, and why only taking one may not be enough to prevent a relapse.

## CHAPTER 17

# What Is Metabolic Syndrome?

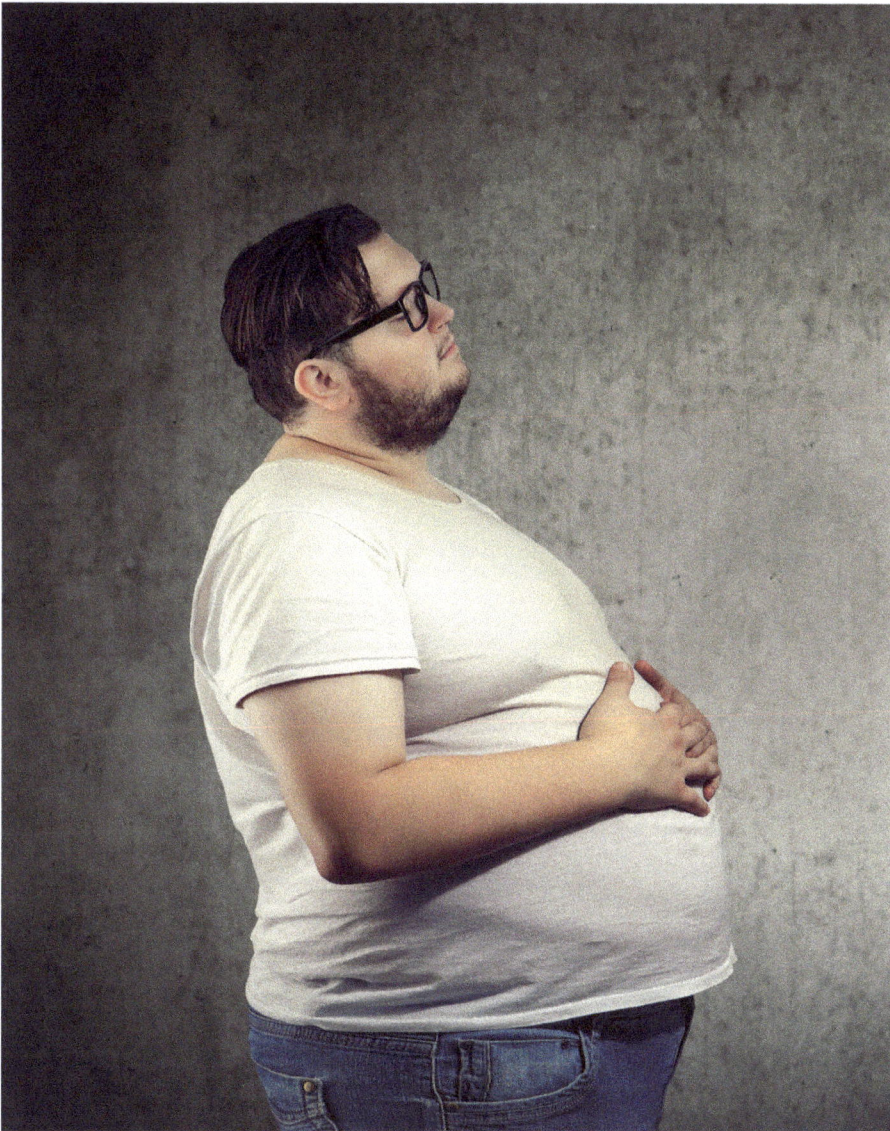

**M**etabolic syndrome is a set of risk factors that increase your risk of heart disease, diabetes, and stroke. It is not itself a disease.

Here are the five risk factors constituting metabolic syndrome.

**FACTOR 1:** A waist circumference of over than 40 inches for men and over 35 inches for women. Measure your waist using a tape measure, at the level of your belly button. Make sure the tape measure is level all the way around. Breathe out, then check the number on the tape measure.

**FACTOR 2:** The second factor is high blood pressure, which is anything greater than 135/85.

**FACTOR 3:** The third is an elevated triglyceride level, which is anything greater than 150 mg/dL. Triglycerides are a type of fat (also called a lipid) used to store unused calories. Unused calories often come from carbohydrates found in sugars and starches. So, after you eat, your body uses the calories from your food to fuel your activities. Unneeded calories are then stored away in the triglycerides.

**Antipsychotic medications increase the risk of developing metabolic syndrome. Some have a higher risk than others.**

# METABOLIC SYNDROME

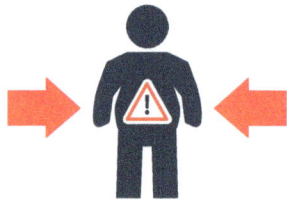

WAIST CIRCUMFERENCE    HIGH BLOOD PRESSURE    HIGH TRIGLYCERIDES    LOW HDL CHOLESTEROL    ELEVATED GLUCOSE LEVEL

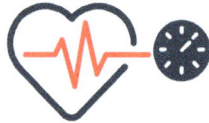

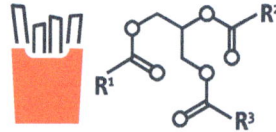

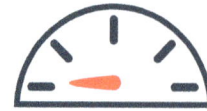

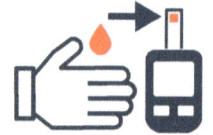

Afterward, your body retrieves some of the triglycerides in between meals and breaks them down for energy.

**FACTOR 4:** The fourth risk factor is low cholesterol in the HDL category. For men, this means HDL cholesterol is less than 40 mg/dL, and for women, it's less than 50 mg/dL. HDL cholesterol isn't the same as total cholesterol. Your cholesterol measurement includes HDL, which is high-density lipoprotein, and LDL, which is low-density lipoprotein. Think of a lipoprotein as a package containing cholesterol and triglycerides. Cholesterol and triglycerides are not soluble in water. To be transported to other parts of your body, they have to attach to a protein escort.

HDL is considered good because it absorbs excess cholesterol and carries it back to the liver for processing. So high levels of HDL lower your risk of heart attack and stroke. This reduced heart attack risk is why having high total cholesterol isn't necessarily bad. It depends on how high it is. But

if you have a high HDL, it's going to raise your total cholesterol. LDL cholesterol is considered bad because it is deposited on artery walls, creating plaques that narrow arteries. These plaques contribute to heart disease and increase the chance of having a stroke. Ideally, you should keep your LDL as low as possible.

**FACTOR 5:** The fifth risk factor is having an elevated fasting blood glucose level, which is anything greater than 100 mg/dL.

Fasting glucose is how much sugar you have in your blood when you haven't eaten anything for at least 8 hours. Insulin is the hormone produced by the pancreas, which processes the glucose from the food you eat.

According to the American Heart Association, you need three out of five of these factors to be diagnosed with metabolic syndrome.

There are only two risk factors that you can detect on your own. You can notice your abdomen getting wider, and you can measure your blood pressure. A 2015 meta-analysis found waist size to be the most useful predictor of metabolic syndrome (Mitchell 2013).

You can also measure your blood pressure. You can't feel your blood pressure rising. Sometimes, if your blood pressure spikes very high, you may feel your head pounding or feel lightheaded. Usually, the only way to know that your blood pressure is elevated is to check it.

## FASTING GLUCOSE LEVELS

| Normal | = | Blood glucose under 100 mg/dL |
|---|---|---|
| Prediabetes | = | Blood glucose of 100–125 mg/dL |
| Diabetes | = | Blood glucose greater than 126 mg/dL |

Blood pressure kits are easy to obtain. You can purchase a reliable digital monitor on Amazon for between $30 and $50. Units that measure blood pressure in the upper arm are generally more reliable than those that measure blood pressure in the wrist.

Your blood pressure fluctuates throughout the day. Suppose you have blood pressure in the borderline range of 130 for the top number or 80–90 for the bottom number. In that case, you should check your blood pressure at different times of day, such as morning and afternoon. Your blood pressure is usually lowest when you're sleeping, and it rises after you wake up. Blood pressure tends to peak in the early afternoon.

The other three factors require blood tests to check your fasting sugar, HDL, and triglycerides. If you're overweight and have high blood pressure, those are signals that you should get your blood levels checked.

## WHAT MAKES THIS HAPPEN?

Obesity is a common cause of metabolic syndrome. Obesity is defined by your body mass index (BMI).

BMI = weight in kilograms/height in meters$^2$

There are handy BMI calculators online, making it easy for you to input your height in feet and inches and your weight in pounds without converting to metric units. One such site is the National Heart, Lung, and Blood Institute. It also has an app you can download to your mobile device.

| BMI RANGES | |
|---|---|
| Normal | 18.5–24. 9 |
| Overweight | 25–29.9 |
| Obese | 30 or greater |

Many things can lead to obesity. But in psychiatry, the antipsychotic medications we use can cause significant weight gain and can lead to metabolic syndrome.

A 2017 article ranked the antipsychotic medications in order of weight-gaining tendency (Dayabandara 2017). The three causing the greatest weight gain were:

- Clozapine
- Olanzapine
- Chlorpromazine.

The next three moderate weight-gaining medications are:

- Quetiapine
- Risperidone
- Paliperidone.

Low on the weight gain scale were:

- Aripiprazole
- Asenapine
- Haloperidol
- Ziprasidone
- Lurasidone.

## HOW CHLORPROMAZINE CHANGED PSYCHIATRY

Chlorpromazine was the first antipsychotic, produced in 1952. It became FDA approved under the brand name Thorazine® in 1957. It transformed psychiatric treatment because it was the first drug to effectively and reliably treat psychosis and mania. It is seen as responsible for deinstitutionalization, a policy beginning in 1955 that moved severely mentally ill people out of large state institutions known as asylums. Part two of the policy involved closing many of these institutions and effectively defunding psychiatric care.

Chlorpromazine is rarely prescribed today because of its side effects. It's markedly sedating in addition to causing significant weight gain. Before chlorpromazine, people who were psychotic, either because of schizophrenia or manic depression (as it was called back then), were committed to institutions where treatment mainly consisted of behavior management without meaningful symptom resolution. So, chlorpromazine allowed these people to regain their sanity.

> **ELEVATED BLOOD PRESSURE AND WEIGHT GAIN OF >10% ARE SIGNALS TO GET BLOOD WORK AND RECONSIDER YOUR MEDICATION.**

Antipsychotics usually cause weight gain by increasing your appetite, especially for carbohydrates and sweets. The increase in appetite isn't a minor one, such as you might experience when watching a movie with friends. Instead, you feel famished, and no amount of eating satisfies your hunger.

Thankfully, this is something you can control if you're aware of it. But many people just don't realize they're eating more. They eat because they're hungry and don't realize they're hungrier than usual.

The sensation to eat is mainly driven by your body's biological need for energy. But here, your hunger is artificially increased. Refusing to yield to the urges to eat won't make

you malnourished. It takes a lot of discipline to hold back, and, with the exercise of sufficient discipline, you can control weight gain.

Antipsychotic-induced weight gain is a big contributor to metabolic syndrome. But some antipsychotics have been shown to interfere with glucose metabolism independent of weight directly.

Studies show the main culprits here are clozapine, olanzapine, and quetiapine.

These three drugs are highly effective but, unfortunately, cause significant weight gain and insulin resistance. This doesn't happen to everyone, but these drugs increase your risk more than the other antipsychotics. So, deciding whether to take one of these medicines involves having you and your doctor undertake a risk-benefit medication analysis. For some, these medications seem almost magical and work better than any of the others.

## WHAT CAN YOU DO ABOUT THIS?

First, knowing about this risk can prompt you to watch your weight.

Sometimes your doctor may put you on one of these medications for a short while. But suppose you're going to take one of these medications for more than six months. In that case, you should make sure you have regular check-ups consisting of, among other things, lab work to monitor lipid and blood sugar levels.

If you gain more than about 10% of your body weight, despite your best efforts to modify your eating habits, you and your doctor should revisit whether you need the medication. For example, with treatment-resistant depression or psychotic depression, we may add aripiprazole for several months to treat symptoms and then taper off the aripiprazole when symptoms improve. Then you would remain only on the antidepressant.

Another option is to add metformin to help you lose weight and improve insulin resistance. The typical weight loss expected after taking metformin is between 5–10% of your weight. True, this isn't huge. Still, it's something. Metformin has a bigger effect on lowering blood sugar when it's elevated.

## CHAPTER 18

# Can you Stop Taking Your Bipolar Medication?

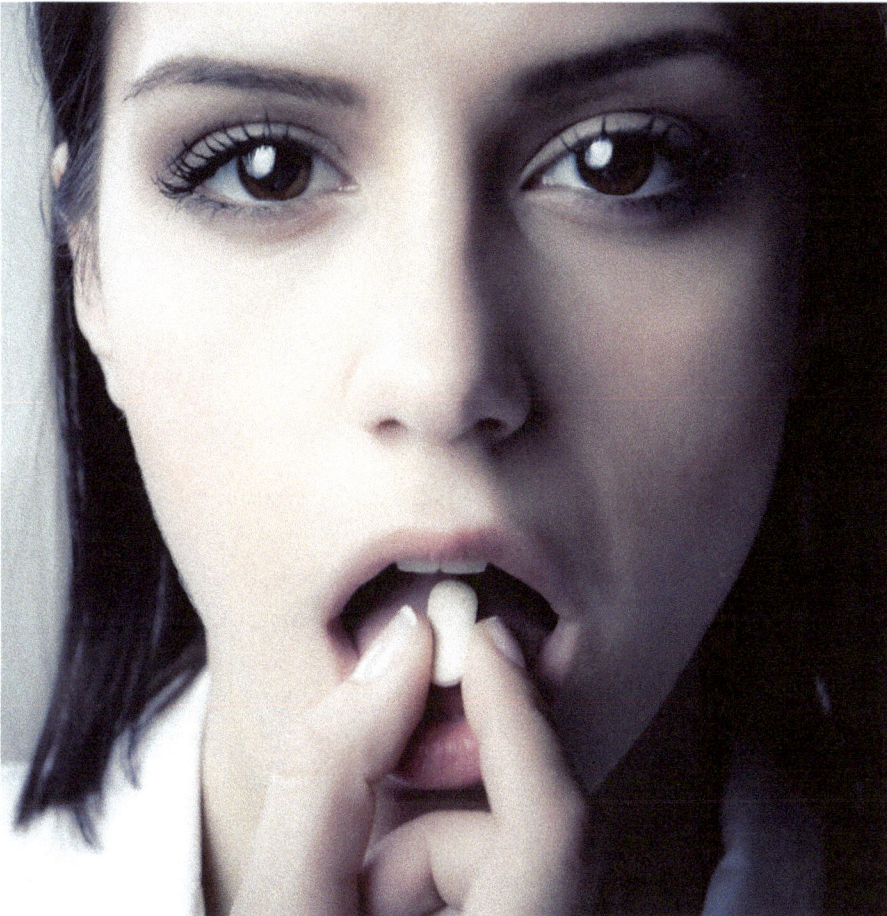

We discussed in Chapter 14 how, with a classical picture of bipolar disorder, you could have periods in between episodes with few to no symptoms. During this period, you're back to normal. Not everyone has the classic picture, however. According to the STEP-BD study, only 58% of people with bipolar disorder types 1 and 2 fully recover (Miklowitz 2007). So, many people still have symptoms in between episodes. The study also showed that 49% had another episode within two years, and twice as many episodes were depression.

If you recover fully between episodes and your episodes are separated by years, you may be able to manage just fine without medication until the next episode.

Bipolar disorder is a serious mental illness that involves recurring episodes of depression and either hypomania or mania. It usually requires medication to treat the acute episodes and prevent their return after they've resolved. But some people go through periods without medication.

IT'S MUCH EASIER TO TWEAK MEDS WHEN YOUR SYMPTOMS CHANGE THAN IT IS TO START NEW AND QUICKLY RAMP UP. SOMETIMES THE SYMPTOMS DON'T RESPOND QUICKLY ENOUGH.

If you choose this strategy to take breaks from your medication between episodes, the success of that plan is based heavily on you being able to recognize early signs of an episode.

Mania can surface quickly and unexpectedly. Often people don't seek help for the mania, especially hypomania, because it can feel good. If you have the more irritable form of hypomania, you might just think you're just going through a rough patch that'll soon pass.

There's a danger associated with watching and waiting.  Once you've sunk into depression or escalated to mania, it's harder to get things under control. It's possible to address this issue with medication, but it's much easier to tweak what you're already on if you have a relapse on medication. But if you're off medication, the process of restarting a medication regimen takes more time. If your doctor tries to do a fast taper upward, you can experience more side effects, like sedation and feeling like a zombie.

Also, if you go too long without medication while you're having an episode, the time you spend in those episodes without treatment makes future episodes harder to treat and less responsive to medication. This is known as "the kindling effect."

Psychotherapy can be a good addition to treatment, but it's not been shown to be effective as the only treatment. But therapy can help delay the onset of future episodes. This additional time can be useful if you're trying to stay off medication in your inter-episode period.

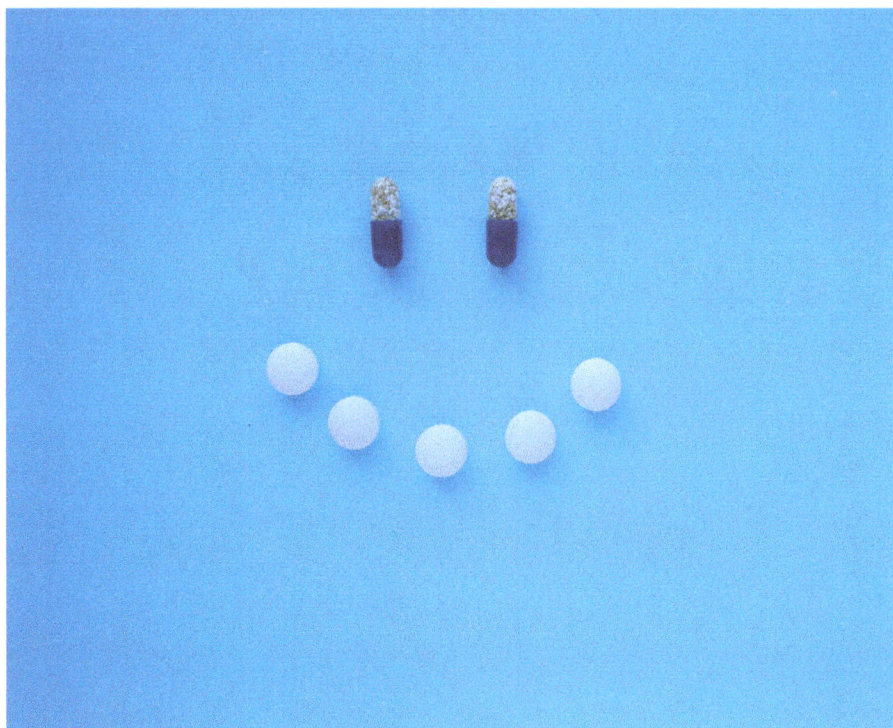

Interpersonal and social rhythm therapy has been shown to be helpful for bipolar disorder. This therapy focuses on problems in your relationships and helps you to establish regular daily routines.

Mania tends to be more destructive interpersonally. In a manic state, you can do all kinds of things that hurt yourself or others, such as having affairs, running up credit cards, ruining business deals, or embarrassing yourself at work or school by acting bizarrely and scaring people. In contrast, depression tends to be more of a silent, personal pain that others don't necessarily see. The people who live with you may see how dysfunctional you are, but they may not appreciate the depth of despair and darkness you experience.

So interpersonal therapy focuses on problematic areas in your life involving how you relate to others in your environment. During therapy, the therapist will help you identify some of these problems and troubleshoot them to find solutions.

We will discuss the social rhythm part of the therapy in the next chapter.

Now let's return to the original question: can people with bipolar disorder stop taking medication? Yes, some can stop for a while. But consistent compliance with medication lowers the odds of your condition worsening over time.  So, although it may be possible to stop your medication, it's not advisable to stop taking medication for this condition.

## CHAPTER 19

# Six Strategies To Manage Bipolar Disorder

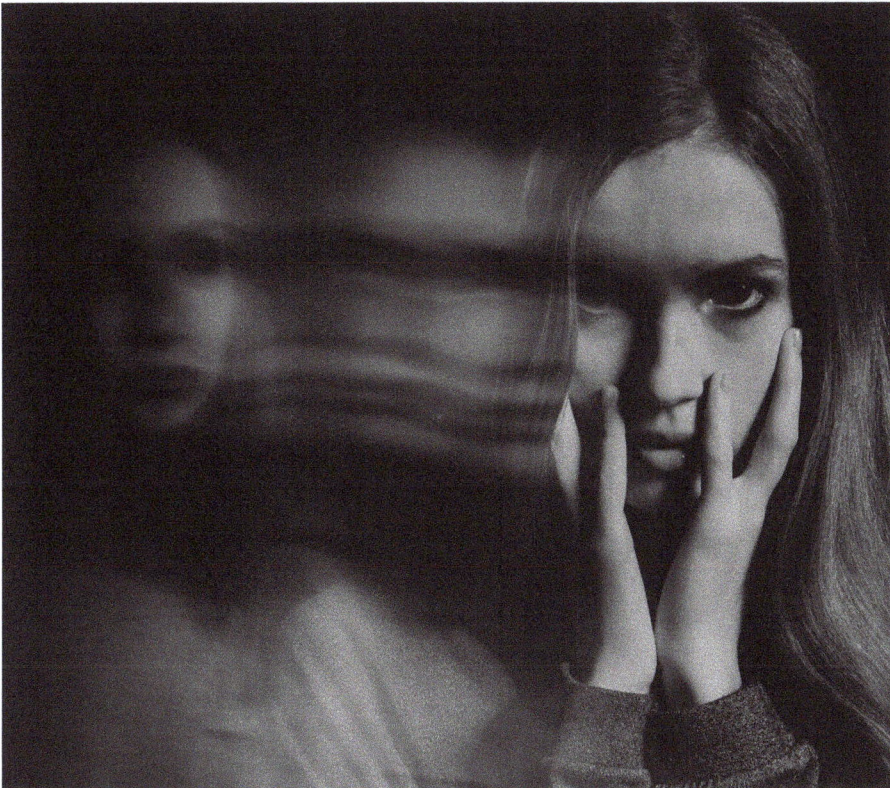

At the end of this chapter, there is a guide summarizing the strategies you can use to track your activities and progress.

## STEP 1: IDENTIFY THINGS THAT TRIGGER AN EPISODE

The trigger can be an episode of depression or mania. Here are some examples:

- Work stress
- Arguments with family members
- Sleeping less
- A change in season, leading to long days and increased light exposure

Chapter 18 addressed why you should stay on medication to manage symptoms and ensure that you remain stable. Even though medication is the mainstay of managing bipolar disorder, there are also ways you can manage bipolar disorder behaviorally, independent of your medication.

> RESEARCH SHOWS THAT STICKING TO A ROUTINE HELPS YOU RECOVER FASTER AND STAY WELL LONGER.

- Change in living situation
- Job loss or promotion
- Illness for you or a family member
- Boredom
- Loneliness
- Substance use (such as marijuana or excess alcohol)
- Financial problems
- Death of family member or close friend
- Anniversary of someone's death.

Write down these triggers so that you can use them in step six.

## STEP 2: KEEP A RECORD OF YOUR MOODS IN A DIARY

You should record your moods as you notice them change or intensify. In a corresponding column, note what's happening when your mood changes or the circumstance related to your mood. Noting the time when your emotion changes can help you see your mood patterns. You can then use this diary to monitor your response to treatments or see when an episode is approaching.

## STEP 3: ESTABLISH A DAILY ROUTINE

Bipolar disorder is highly sensitive to changes in your body clock and overall body homeostasis.  You can think of this as your body's overall rhythm. An early sign of a manic episode approaching is a decreased need for sleep. Research shows that social and interpersonal rhythm therapy

helps you recover faster and lengthens the time in between episodes.

Your schedule may not be entirely under your control. But adjusting your life to eat and sleep at the same time each day improves your overall health.

Keeping a regular schedule doesn't mean you have to eat three meals a day. The key is eating your meals, regardless of how many you eat, around the same time. People using this therapy may use the Social Rhythm Metric (SRM) to track their activities. There's a 17-item form and a shorter 5-item form.

With the SRM-5, you track the following items:

- Get out of bed
- Have the first contact with another person
- Start work, housework, or volunteer activities
- Eat dinner
- Go to bed.

This metric aims to set these activities as anchor points and track the times for at least two weeks. The goal is to keep them as constant as you can. Sometimes maintaining your schedule doesn't work. That's okay. But if you aim to work around these anchor points each day, you're likely to keep some of

## WITH THE SRM-5, YOU TRACK THE FOLLOWING ITEMS:

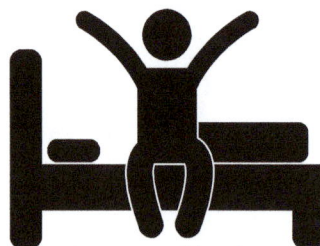

Get out of bed

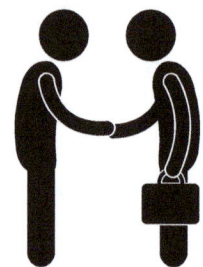

Have the first contact with another person

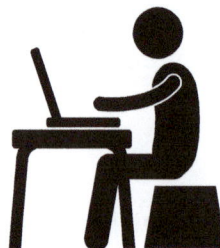

Start work, housework, or volunteer activities

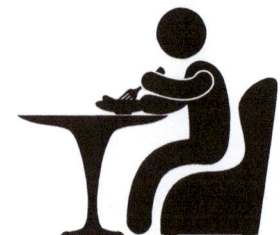

Eat dinner

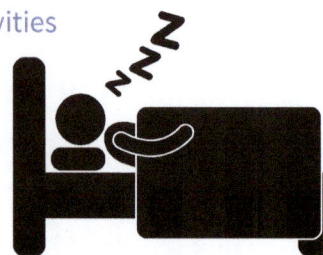

Go to bed

them consistent over the week, even if you can't do all five every day. Averaging several points a day over the week is better than having an unstructured, free-flowing schedule.

## STEP 4: CREATE AN ACTIVITY PLAN

You'll use this when you're oversleeping or withdrawing during your depressed phase. It's like having a disaster management plan in place before a storm comes.

Let's consider this scenario. When you're feeling well, your usual sleep time is 11 pm to 6 am. But when you get depressed, you start going to bed around 9 pm, and you may sleep until 8 am or 9 am. These extended sleep hours will only work if you have a flexible job or school schedule that allows you to wake up when you want.

You'll notice your sleep times are changing if you're keeping up with your daily rhythm from step 3. When you start slipping into this extended schedule, pull out your activity plan to see your everyday activities. Some examples may be getting up to walk the dog, taking a walk around the neighborhood, driving to the library, vacuuming the house, etc. They should be simple activities that you can slog through in your depressed state. It still benefits you to keep your body moving. This process of getting moving is called "behavioral activation therapy." It's more complicated than this, but this is just one example.

## STEP 5: USE DARK THERAPY FOR MANIC EPISODES

Typically, during a manic or hypomanic episode, you need

Blue light refers to the wavelength of light in the visible light spectrum. What we see as white light is a mixture of different wavelengths of light. The other colors, in order of longest to shortest wavelength, are:

Red → Orange → Yellow → Green → Blue → Indigo → Violet

Red light has a wavelength of around 700 nanometers, and violet has a wavelength of around 380 nanometers. Blue light corresponds to a wavelength of 480 nanometers. You can see these individual colors if you view the light through a prism. You can also see these colors as an optical illusion when they're refracted through water droplets and form a rainbow.

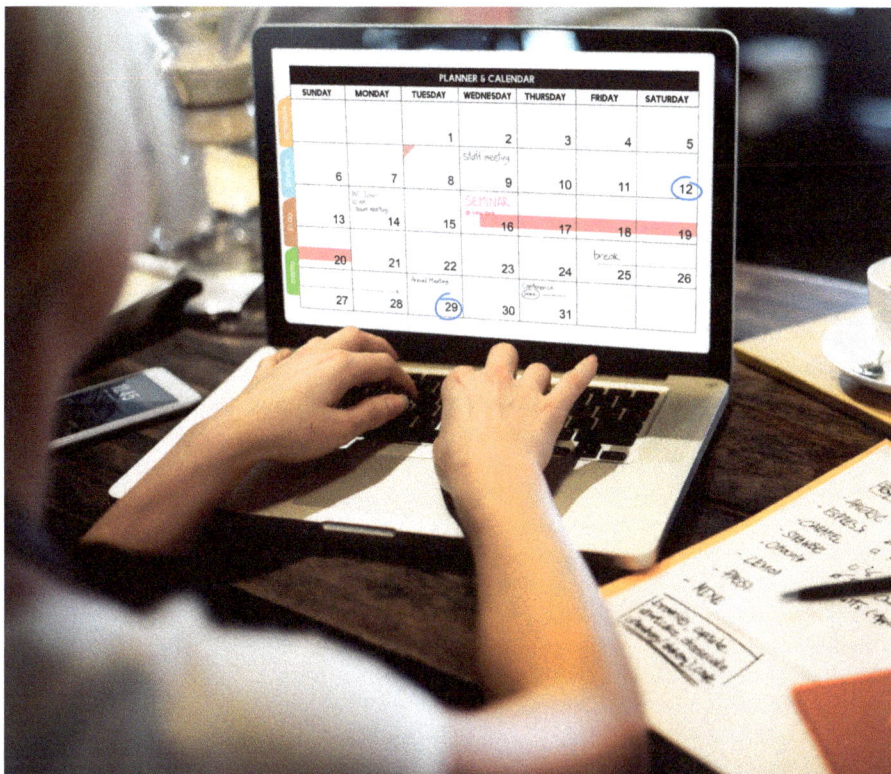

less sleep. Some people may only sleep a couple of hours and feel fine. Others can go a day or two without sleeping at all. But sleep deprivation fuels mania and makes it ramp up to where it's out of control.

Dark therapy works by blocking blue light from sunlight, house lights, and digital devices. It fools the body into thinking it's nighttime, enabling you to sleep.

Blue light blocks the release of melatonin. Melatonin is a

hormone secreted in the brain to signal to your body that it's dark. Light, especially blue light, turns off melatonin production. The absence of melatonin is a signal to your body that it's daytime and, therefore, time to be awake. When the sun goes down, or you put on the glasses, your body releases melatonin, and your body thinks it's nighttime.

Dark therapy uses blue light blocking glasses in the evening to simulate darkness and train your body clock to recognize a consistent pattern of night and day. The glasses have an orange lens, which is the opposite color to blue on a traditional color wheel. These orange lenses negate the blue light you see.

## WHY DOES THIS WORK?

Your eyes have a photoreceptor containing a pigment called melanopsin. These melanopsin receptors detect light, not images. You have a separate pathway to detect images through your primary vision, and those nerve cells connect to your visual cortex. The melanopsin receptors connect to the suprachiasmatic nucleus, which is responsible for controlling your biological clock. Your suprachiasmatic nucleus communicates with the pineal gland to secrete melatonin.

Melanopsin photoreceptors are selectively sensitive to short-wavelength light, like blue light.

Blue light activates the receptor and causes the pineal gland to stop producing melatonin. When you're exposed to daylight and blue light from devices, your melatonin is shut off or greatly reduced. When the blue light is blocked, these receptors are deactivated, and melatonin is released.

Here's how the glasses fit into this matrix. The blue light blocking glasses have an amber-colored lens which blocks out the blue light you otherwise see. It feels as if you're walking around in complete darkness when you wear the glasses because your light detection receptors aren't activated. Visually, you still see the light, but because the receptors aren't detecting light, your brain thinks you're in darkness. When your brain "sees" darkness, melatonin is released. So, the blue light blocking glasses are a way to manipulate night and day to secure a consistent circadian rhythm and sleep schedule.

The protocol for dark therapy during a manic episode is to wear the glasses from 6 pm to 8 am. If you work late, you should wear them in your work setting (if appropriate). Wearing them in the early evening becomes even more important in the spring and summer, when days are longer. You don't need to wear the glasses while you're sleeping. You would put them on at 6 pm, then take them off when you get in bed and turn off the lights. If your bedroom isn't completely dark, you can use an eye mask to block

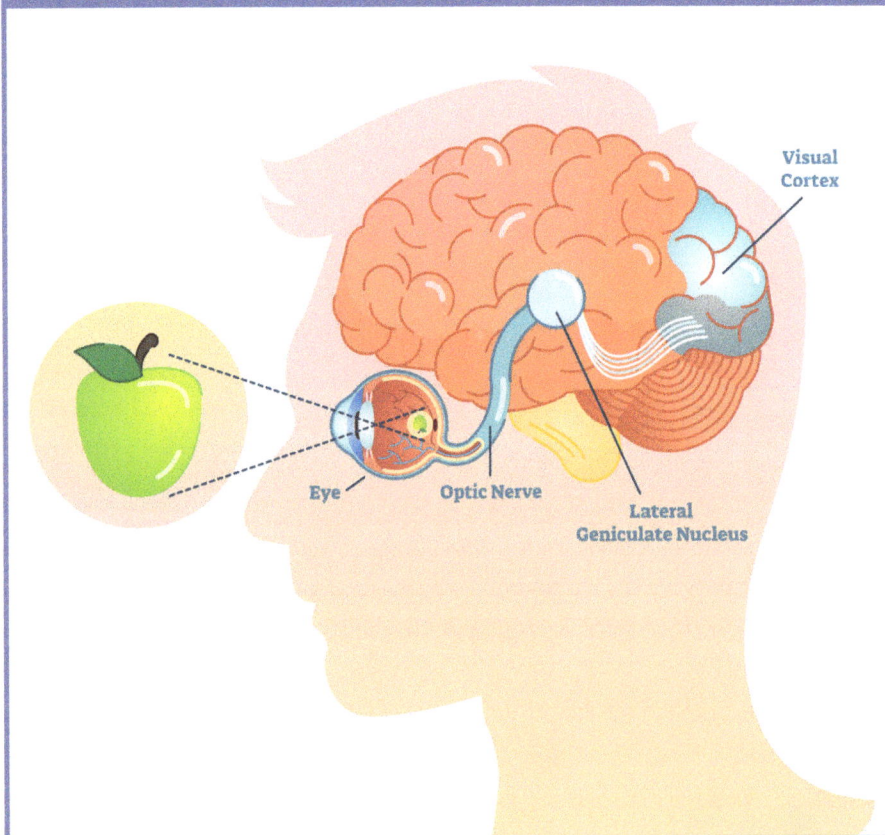

## HOW THE EYE WORKS

Visual Cortex

Eye

Optic Nerve

Lateral Geniculate Nucleus

the light instead of wearing the glasses.

During summer, when it's light until 8–9 pm, you may need to wear the glasses when driving home from work or doing yard work. But don't start wearing the glasses earlier than 6 pm because doing so can disrupt your circadian rhythm and worsen your mood. It's important to remember that your body is fooled into believing that you're walking around in the dark while you're wearing them. You don't want your body to think you're in the dark all day and all night. And, by the way, the glasses don't make you sleepy, at least not immediately. But they help restore your sleep schedule, so you're back to sleeping soundly in the evening.

Once your mania resolves, you can still wear the glasses as a maintenance measure, providing you're not depressed and sleeping longer than 9 hours. During the maintenance phase, you can push back when you start wearing them from 6 pm to between 8 and 10 pm.

The use of these glasses has been studied in people who do not have bipolar disorder but have trouble falling asleep. One study showed improved sleep in people who wore the glasses about 2 hours before bedtime.

Uvex Skyper glasses have been used in some studies: you can buy these on Amazon. For a list of recommended resources, visit

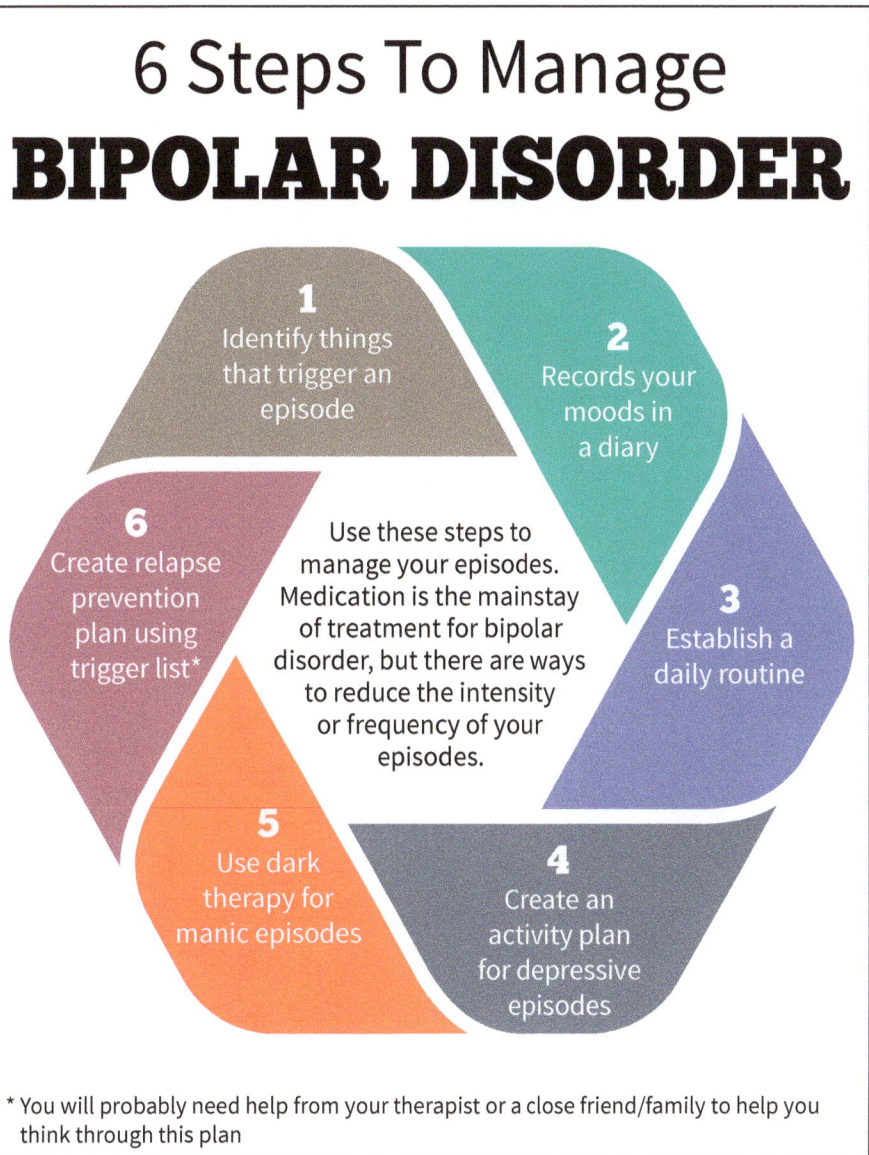

# 6 Steps To Manage
# BIPOLAR DISORDER

1 Identify things that trigger an episode

2 Records your moods in a diary

3 Establish a daily routine

4 Create an activity plan for depressive episodes

5 Use dark therapy for manic episodes

6 Create relapse prevention plan using trigger list*

Use these steps to manage your episodes. Medication is the mainstay of treatment for bipolar disorder, but there are ways to reduce the intensity or frequency of your episodes.

* You will probably need help from your therapist or a close friend/family to help you think through this plan

https://Markspsychiatry.com/resources.

## STEP 6: CREATE A RELAPSE PREVENTION PLAN

This step is where you pull out your list of triggers from step 1. You may need help from your doctor or therapist in creating this plan. A close friend or relative familiar with your situation can also help you brainstorm ideas.

Go through your trigger list and create strategies to help avoid the triggers altogether or help you become less reactive to them. This won't guarantee that you'll never have another episode, but it might make a difference to the severity of the episode or even its timing. Bipolar disorder is a biological illness; it's not solely dependent on stress or trigger factors. But you can try to reduce the number of episodes and their severity by controlling your triggers.

Download the worksheets: https://markspsychiatry.com/handbook-sheets

# RELAPSE PREVENTION PLAN

## INSTRUCTIONS

Record situations that upset or aggravate you in a way. Then write down your reactions to these situations. In the relapse prevention section, you will evaluate these triggers to see how you can avoid them or lessen their impact.

## TRIGGER LIST

### SAMPLE TRIGGERS

Staying up too late on my phone

Drinking too much

Not taking a break on the weekends

Waiting too late to finish assignments

Letting my partner irritate me

Going to too many parties in a week

| Trigger | Reaction |
| --- | --- |
| | |
| | |
| | |
| | |

| Trigger | Reaction |
|---|---|
|  |  |
|  |  |
|  |  |
|  |  |
|  |  |
|  |  |
|  |  |

# RELAPSE PREVENTION PLAN

## INTERVENTION PLAN

Look at each situation on your trigger list. Think about what role these triggers played in the lead-up to a depressive or manic/hypomanic episode. Brainstorm how to avoid the situation or lessen the impact of the situation and write down your ideas.

| Situation | Intervention |
|---|---|
|  |  |
|  |  |
|  |  |
|  |  |
|  |  |

# ACTIVITY PLAN

## INSTRUCTIONS

Maintaining a routine is very important with bipolar disorder. Even minor disruptions to your routine can make you more vulnerable to becoming unstable and can trigger an episode.

## STEP ONE

Establish your **anchor points**. These are the times you wake up, go to bed and eat your meals. You can use a short range for your meal times.

Wake up _____

Go to bed _____

Breakfast _____

Lunch _____

Dinner _____

## STEP TWO

Have a backup plan for activities to implement when you are depressed and oversleeping or lying around with little energy or motivation. This is a plan to force structure into your day. *This can also address withdrawing from people.*

## ACTIVITY OPTIONS

| | |
|---|---|
| 1 | |
| 2 | |
| 3 | |
| 4 | |
| 5 | |
| 6 | |
| 7 | |
| 8 | |
| 9 | |

# ACTIVITY PLAN

SAMPLE

## INSTRUCTIONS

Maintaining a routine is very important with bipolar disorder. Even minor disruptions to your routine can make you more vulnerable to becoming unstable and can trigger an episode.

## STEP ONE

Establish your **anchor points**. These are the times you wake up, go to bed and eat your meals. You can use a short range for your meal times.

| | | | |
|---|---|---|---|
| Wake up | 7am | Breakfast | 7:30–8am |
| Go to bed | 11pm | Lunch | 12pm–1:30pm |
| | | Dinner | 6pm–7:30pm |

## STEP TWO

Have a backup plan for activities to implement when you are depressed and oversleeping or lying around with little energy or motivation. This is a plan to force structure into your day. ***This can also address withdrawing from people.***

### ACTIVITY OPTIONS

| | |
|---|---|
| 1 | Walk around the block |
| 2 | Drive to Walmart and look at the electronics |
| 3 | Go to Starbucks with my laptop on Saturday for 1 hour in the morning |
| 4 | Meet up with my sister for lunch |
| 5 | Go to the library and sit in the media section for 30 minutes |
| 6 | Fill one box with stuff from the basement and donate it to Goodwill |
| 7 | Take three pictures outside and post them on Instagram |
| 8 | |
| 9 | |

# MOOD DIARY

## INSTRUCTIONS

Record your moods as you feel them intensify. You can also track unusual moods that may be a sign that something is changing.

## SAMPLE MOODS

Happy, sad, tired, excited, anxious, fearful, worried, angry, depressed, hopeless, tense, ambitious, invincible, rageful

| Time | Mood | What Was Happening? |
|---|---|---|
| 8am–10am | | |
| 10am–12pm | | |
| 12pm–2pm | | |
| 2pm–4pm | | |
| 4pm–6pm | | |
| 6pm–8pm | | |
| 8pm–10pm | | |
| 10pm–12am | | |
| 12am–2am | | |
| 2am–4am | | |
| 4am–6am | | |
| 6am–8am | | |

## CHAPTER 20

# Bright Light Therapy For Bipolar Depression

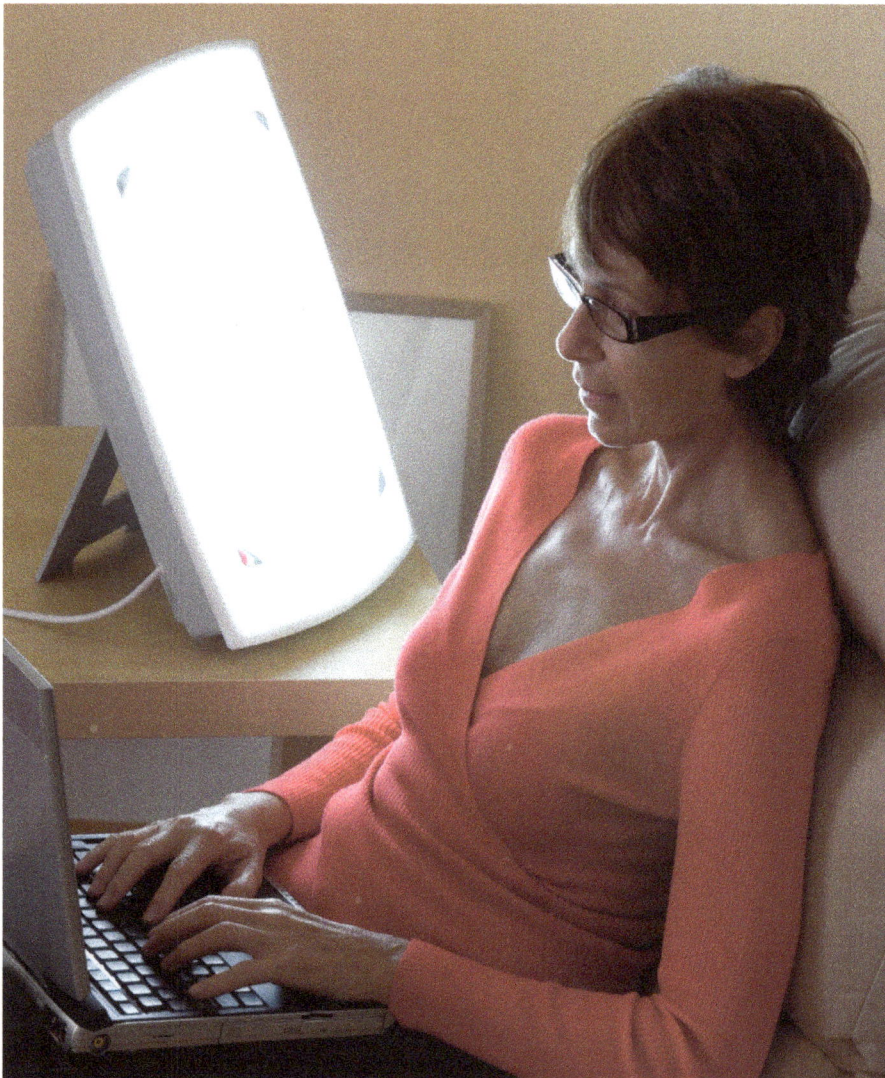

**P**eople with bipolar depression had to be cautious about using the early morning light therapy because of the risk of the light triggering a manic episode.

After more research in this area, a protocol was developed using bright light therapy to treat bipolar depression. As tempting as it is to use antidepressants during the depression phase, they destabilize bipolar disorder. Bright light therapy is a good non-medication option for treating depressive episodes.

Here's how the therapy works.

With bipolar depression, you should use the light in the middle of the day, between noon and

Light therapy has been used to treat unipolar depression and seasonal affective disorder (SAD). The protocol consists of using blue light or bright light boxes early in the morning.

LIGHT THERAPY FOR BIPOLAR DEPRESSION CAN BE A CONVENIENT WAY TO ADDRESS DEPRESSION WITHOUT TAKING MORE MEDICATION.

> YOU SHOULD REMAIN ON YOUR MOOD STABILIZER WHILE USING LIGHT THERAPY.

2 pm. You should start with a 15-minute timeframe and increase this time by 15 minutes every week to a maximum of 60 minutes. This protocol is different from light therapy for unipolar depression, where you start with a 30-minute timeframe. Moving slower reduces the risk of destabilizing your mood. But because you're going slower, it may take longer to see an improvement.

You can buy small lights that conveniently fit in the palm of your hand. But to be effective, a light should have a large surface area, like 12 inches by 17 inches, and it needs to produce 10,000 lux of bright white light. This intensity is generated at the light box and drops off as you move away from it. At two feet away, your eyes experience roughly 2,000–3,000 lux.

The light box selected should emit full spectrum white light with a UV filter.

## POSITIONING

It's best to sit with the light above you and about 1–2 feet away. The light should be at about a 45-degree angle from your face, preferably above your head. Don't stare directly at it. You can do other things, like read or eat, while using the light. Just make sure you don't have your head down so low that the light misses your eyes.

## HOW LONG SHOULD YOU USE BRIGHT LIGHT THERAPY?

If you respond to bright light therapy, it's reasonable to continue it for 12 months after your depression resolves. Continuing in this manner is like continuing antidepressant therapy for a year. In the maintenance phase, you may be able to get by using it three times a week. But if you notice your depression symptoms start to return, go back to using it daily.

## CAN YOU GET THE SAME EFFECT BY GOING OUTSIDE OR LOOKING OUT OF A WINDOW?

It depends. The table below compares the different kinds of light.

In theory, if you don't have a 10,000-lux light box, you could get the same effect by exposing yourself to bright outdoor light as long as clouds or trees do not block the light. Sun shining through a window may be the equivalent of indoor light if the sun's rays are shining directly through the window.

You should remain on your regular medication for bipolar disorder. If you've stopped taking your mood stabilizers, you're at risk of switching into hypomania or mania if you use light therapy as your only method of treatment. This therapy is designed for use during the depressed phase of your bipolar disorder, as an alternative to using an antidepressant to treat depression. If your doctor has you on an antidepressant with a mood stabilizer and you're still depressed, you can use light therapy, but watch out for hypomania. If you notice you feel better after only 15 minutes of light therapy, then there's no need to increase the exposure to 60 minutes. Just stick with the 15 minutes.

| | |
|---|---|
| Direct sunlight without clouds: | 32,000–100,000 lux |
| Ambient daylight (mix of direct and indirect sunlight): | 10,000–25,000 lux |
| Overcast daylight: | 1,000 lux |
| Sunrise/sunset: | 400 lux |
| Indoor light: | 100–200 lux |
| Indoor light at night: | 40 lux |

## ADVERSE EFFECTS

Bright light therapy has few serious side effects. But the most common ones include headache, eye strain, nausea, and agitation. Adverse effects are not permanent and tend to resolve either by decreasing the light exposure time or discontinuing the treatment altogether.

With bright light therapy, more is not always better. Keep the light exposure to what you need: don't exceed 60 minutes. If you notice a meaningful improvement, don't try to do more of it in the late afternoon or evening. It can delay the time you fall asleep.

## WHY WOULDN'T EVERYONE USE LIGHT THERAPY?

There are some practical barriers to treatment. You have to buy the device, and your insurance may not cover its cost. But it's a one-time cost, and some of the lights are under $100. Perhaps a greater barrier is the time and discipline required. If you need 60 minutes to see an effect, this will consume a chunk of your day. That means you need the kind of job or school schedule where you can get an hour to yourself undisturbed, with privacy. If you can get past these barriers, it can be an effective way to manage depression.

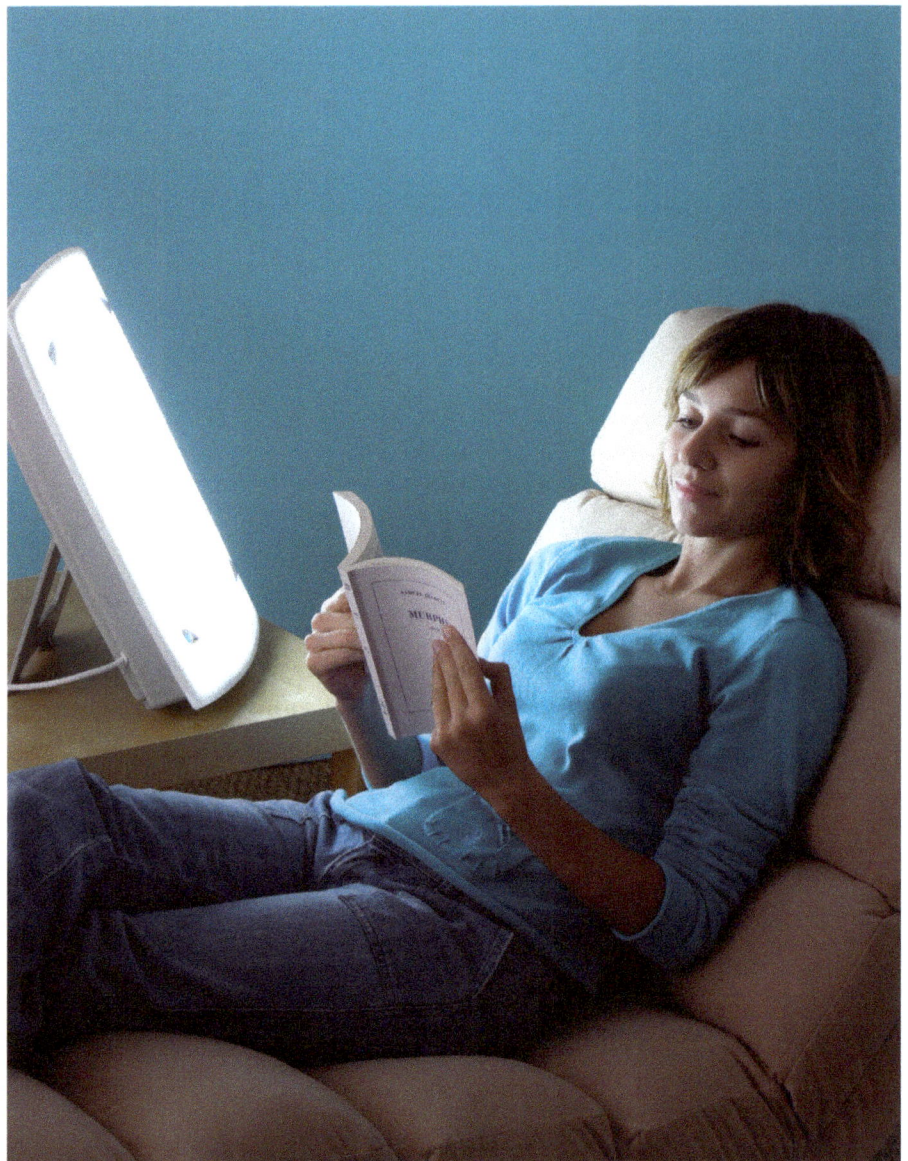

## CHAPTER 21

# Watch Out For Springtime Mania

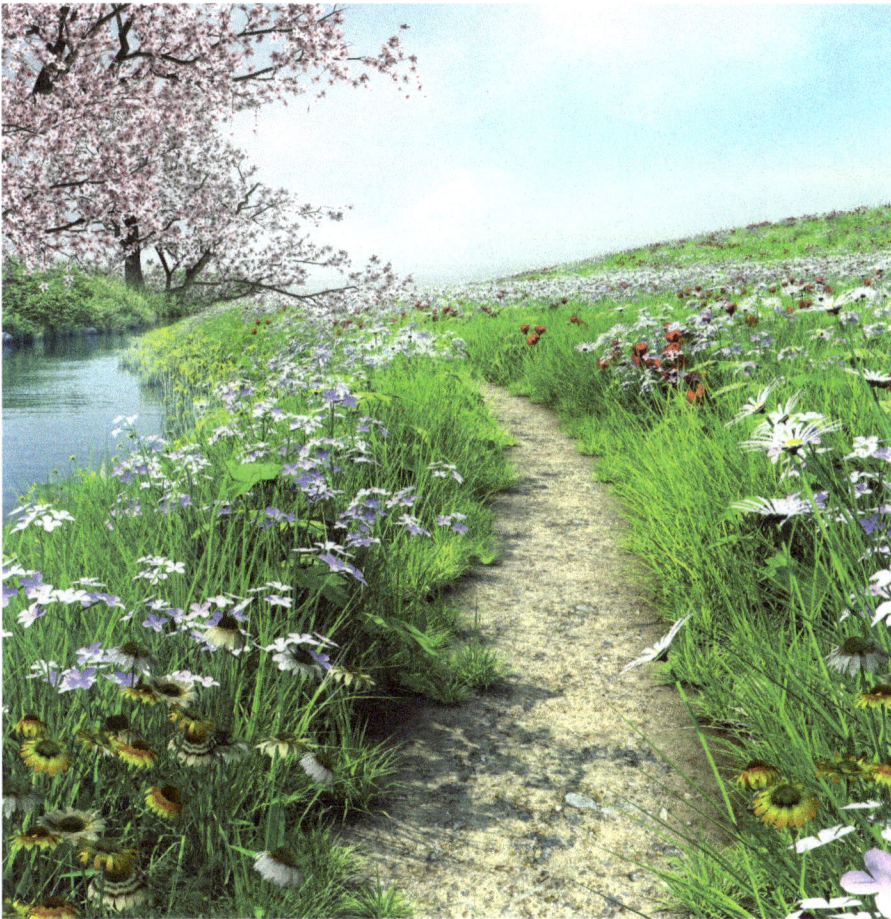

Here's how the longer days can impact you negatively. Longer days translate into engaging in more evening activities that may not end until, say, 9 pm. Then it takes longer to settle down in the evening. Before you know it, you're staying up later and getting less sleep. Reduced sleep promotes mania.

Let's review how the seasons work in the northern hemisphere.

In December, we have the winter solstice. This is the shortest day of the year and the longest night. Typically, that falls around December 21 or 22. Then, as we go through the winter into January and February, the days lengthen, and the nights get shorter. When we get to March, we have the spring equinox, when

As we move from winter to spring and into summer, we get longer days and more sunlight exposure. As such, you may notice your mood ramping up. This rapid change in light, not the extent of exposure to it, makes the biggest difference in triggering mania or hypomania.

PEOPLE WITH BIPOLAR DISORDER ARE VERY SENSITIVE TO CHANGES IN CIRCADIAN RHYTHM.

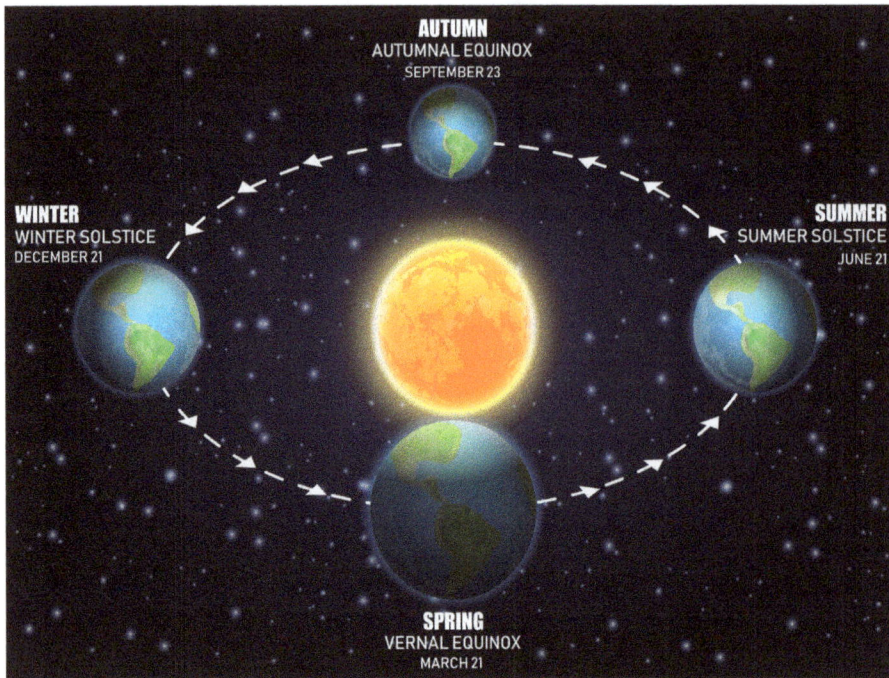

you feel hungry and when your energy rises and falls. So, if your body clock gets thrown off, you can feel hungry at odd hours, and you have energy when you shouldn't be energetic, such as in the middle of the night.

The rate of change in sunlight varies according to where you live. In the United States, sunlight increases most rapidly in the Sunbelt, Northwest, and Northern Midwest. So, if you live in these areas, you should pay close attention to changes in your mood and activity level in March and April.

there is an equal amount of day and night. This usually occurs around March 20.

From there, the days get longer and longer until you reach the summer solstice in June: the longest day of the year and the shortest period of nighttime. Then the nights stretch out and become longer until you reach the fall equinox in September. Then you have an equal amount of day and night again. After the fall equinox, the days get shorter until you reach the winter solstice in December. Then the cycle starts all over again.

These differences in day and night are greatest as you get further

away from the equator. So, the winter solstice in parts of Alaska means having 24 hours of night. For example, Barrow, Alaska, in the Arctic Circle, experiences 67 days of darkness from November to January and 80 days of straight daylight in June and July.

## HOW DOES ALL THIS RELATE TO MANIA?

People with bipolar disorder can be highly sensitive to circadian rhythm changes or changes in the body clock. Some are more sensitive than others. Light is a powerful trigger affecting your circadian rhythm. Your circadian rhythm not only controls when you sleep but also affects when

What can you do about this?

**1** Recognize signs that you may be becoming manic. Typical signs are things such as having irregular sleep, pressured speech, and lots of activity.

**2** Adhere to a strict routine from February through May if you're in the northern hemisphere and September to December if you're in the southern hemisphere.

**3** Wear blue light blocking glasses 1–2 hours before bedtime during springtime as maintenance, even when you're not having manic symptoms.

# COMPARISON OF SIMILAR CONDITIONS

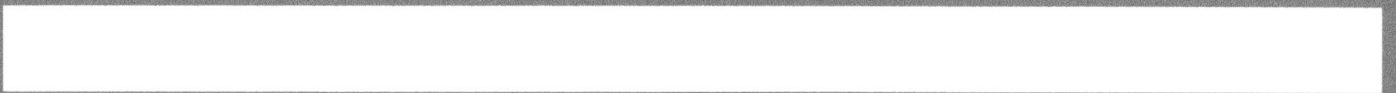

## CHAPTER 22

# Bipolar vs. Borderline Personality Disorder

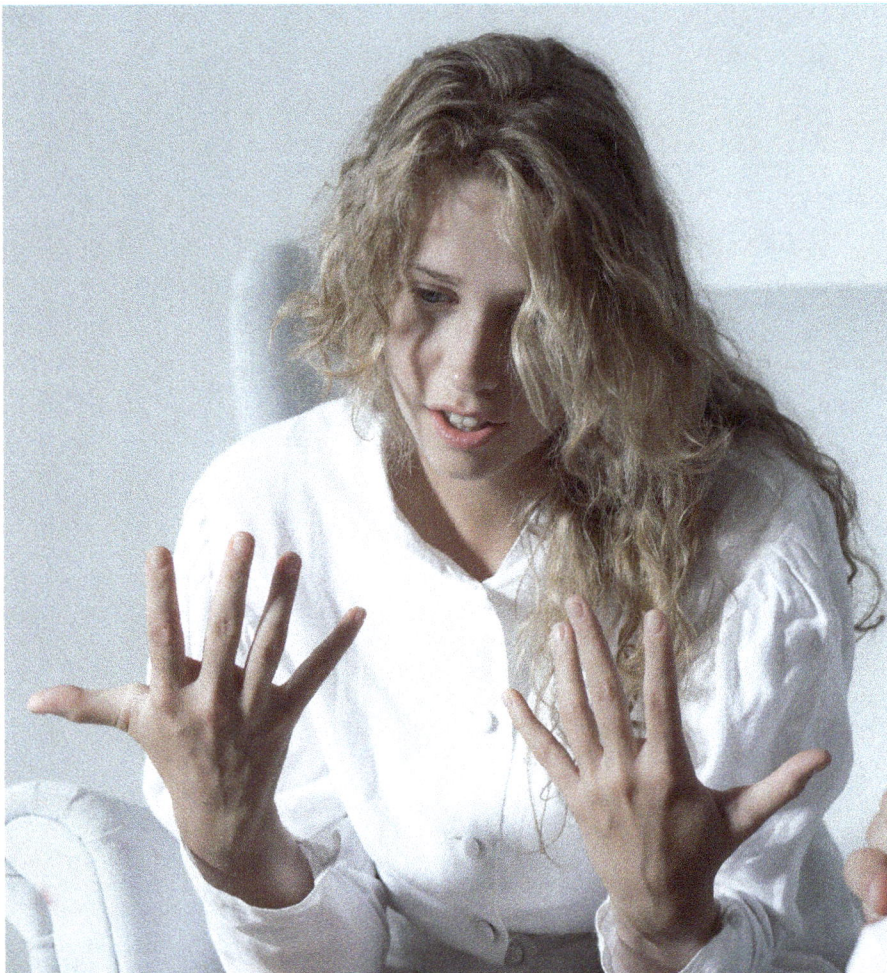

Another analogy would be comparing your personality to a region's climate, and your mood to the current weather. The climate remains stable, but the weather can frequently change.

A person with narcissistic personality disorder who gets depressed will look different from a person with dependent personality disorder who becomes depressed. The narcissistic person, because of their self-centeredness, may look angry and self-loathing. In contrast, the dependent person can become more pitiful and helpless because of their neediness. These are broad-stroke examples.

Here's how the *Diagnostic Manual* defines borderline personality disorder.

There is a notable difference between personality disorders and psychiatric illnesses like depression, anxiety, or bipolar disorder. Your personality is a measure of your hardwiring, whereas an illness concerns your state at the time.

THE PRIMARY TREATMENT FOR BORDERLINE PERSONALITY IS THERAPY, WITH OR WITHOUT MEDICATION.

"A pattern of unstable relationships, self-image, and emotional expression, and marked impulsivity, beginning by early adulthood and present in a variety of contexts, as indicated by five (or more) of the following:"

## BORDERLINE PERSONALITY DISORDER

**1** Frantic efforts to avoid real or imagined abandonment

**2** A pattern of unstable and intense interpersonal relationships

**3** Identity disturbance: markedly and persistently unstable self-image or sense of self

**4** Impulsivity in at least two areas that are potentially self-damaging

**5** Recurrent suicidal behavior, gestures, or threats, or self-mutilating behavior

**6** Unstable, reactive mood

**7** Chronic feelings of emptiness

**8** Inappropriate, intense anger or difficulty controlling anger

**9** Transient, stress-related paranoid ideation or severe dissociative symptoms

### 1. Frantic efforts to avoid real or imagined abandonment

An example of this would be reading too much into things. Things you say are interpreted to mean that you're finished with the person or that you're abandoning them in some way.

### 2. A pattern of unstable and intense interpersonal relationships

An example of this is alternating between extremes of idealization and devaluation.

In this kind of relationship, the person with borderline personality disorder may at one point think you're the best thing ever (idealization). You can do nothing wrong. Then, in the next moment or next day, they see you as the worst person in the entire universe (devaluation).

### 3. Identity disturbance: markedly and persistently unstable self-image or sense of self

This kind of identity disturbance occurs at a deep level. It's not being confused about whether you're meant to be a teacher or an astronaut. Instead, it has to do with confusion about core identity issues, like gender, sexuality, or spirituality.

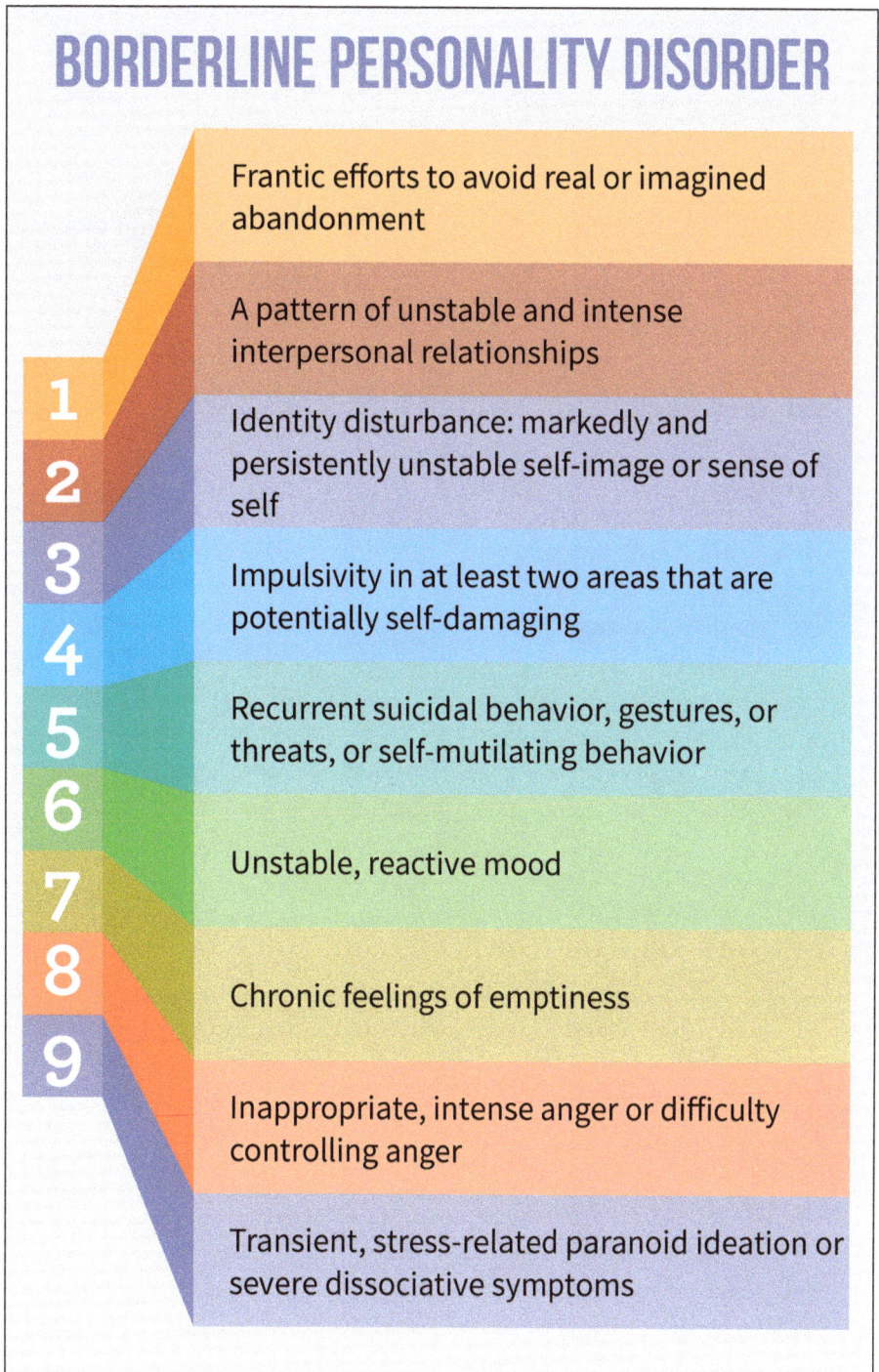

### 4. Impulsivity in at least two areas that are potentially self-damaging

Some examples of this could be reckless spending, reckless sexuality, drug abuse, or binge eating.

### 5. Recurrent suicidal behavior, gestures, or threats, or self-mutilating behavior

This includes behaviors such as cutting yourself or taking an overdose of pills. You don't want to die; you are responding to internal distress.

**6. Unstable, reactive mood**

Examples of this would be episodic low mood, irritability, or anxiety, usually lasting several hours and rarely more than a few days. These rapid mood shifts are one of the key differences between borderline personality disorder and bipolar disorder.

**7. Chronic feelings of emptiness**

This is one of the reasons people with borderline personality disorder cut themselves. It's a coping mechanism to help them feel real. Also, some people cut themselves to relieve tension.

**8. Inappropriate, intense anger or difficulty controlling anger**

This can look like temper tantrums, constant anger, or physical fights.

**9. Transient, stress-related paranoid ideation or severe dissociative symptoms**

Clinicians sometimes call these micro psychotic episodes. They're not full-blown psychosis, but they're close to it.

To diagnose borderline personality disorder, you must have at least five of those characteristics or behaviors occurring around the same time. If you have less than five, you may have borderline traits or features, but you do not have the disorder. For example, suppose you cut yourself from time to time when you get frustrated. That's the only poor coping skill you use. In that case, you wouldn't be diagnosed with borderline personality disorder based on that one feature.

Borderline personality disorder looks similar to bipolar disorder because mood swings and impulsivity are common to both. But with borderline personality disorder, you're more likely to have mood swings from hour to hour or over the day.

With bipolar disorder, the group of symptoms making up an episode needs to last two weeks if you're depressed and one week if you're manic. You aren't shifting in and out of the states from hour to hour. Also, a fear of abandonment and unstable self-identity have more to do with your hardwiring. Your environment can also influence these issues. It's essentially the nature versus nurture issue: how much of who you are is based on genes and how you were raised in your formative years. These issues are independent of bipolar disorder. Think of mania like a storm that swoops in, creates significant damage, then swoops out, leaving the hot climate behind.

Another example of the practical difference between the two disorders is how you manage conflict and distress. If you get depressed, the coping skills you employ are a product of your personality, not the depression itself. The depression may push you into doing something that's self-harming. But it's your personality that reacts to the depression with self-harm.

Treatments for borderline personality disorder and bipolar disorder are different but overlap. The primary treatment for borderline personality disorder is a psychotherapy called dialectical behavioral therapy or DBT. It's an offshoot of cognitive behavior therapy developed specifically for borderline personality disorder. It's highly effective when implemented by someone trained in DBT, and usually conducted as a combination of individual and group skill learning sessions. Other psychotherapies used for borderline personality disorder are schema-focused therapy, mentalization-based therapy, and transference-focused therapy.

## DISSOCIATION

Dissociation happens when a person disconnects from their present situation. This disconnection can be from the current environment, your thoughts, or even from yourself. Sometimes this can result from repeated physical or sexual abuse, especially when it occurs in childhood. One way you cope with the trauma is to mentally pull away as if it's not happening to you. You can mentally take yourself to another place while the trauma is happening to you. With borderline personality disorder, this dissociation happens frequently.

If someone with borderline personality disorder also becomes depressed, they may require medication to get through the depression. Also, sometimes the swinging moods one can experience with borderline personality disorder can respond well to mood stabilizers even though it's not considered bipolar disorder. Mood stabilizers stabilize your mood regardless of what make your mood unstable. They can be particularly helpful in treating mood shifts or intense anger from the personality disorder.

## COMBINATION OF BORDERLINE PERSONALITY AND BIPOLAR DISORDER

People with borderline personality disorder can also have bipolar disorder. Some refer to this as borderpolar (which isn't an official term).

Studies show that about 20% of people have both disorders.

The disorders occurring together complicate the course of the illness. The combination tends to produce the following:

- Increased mood swings (which means less time feeling stable, despite being on a good medication regimen)
- Earlier age of onset of bipolar disorder
- Increased suicidality, either in attempts or thoughts
- Increased aggression and hostility
- Increased substance misuse
- Increased comorbid diagnoses (which means co-occurring illnesses, such as PTSD and OCD)
- Increased instances of unemployment and hospitalizations.

## WHAT DOES HAVING BOTH LOOK LIKE?

You have episodes of depression and mania that come and go and experience distress, sadness, or dissatisfaction with life that doesn't change even when your depression or mania has passed. Determining whether your depression or mania has passed is difficult when you're still feeling emotionally unstable.

That can lead to overmedication.

Also, borderline personality disorder is often accompanied by fears of being rejected or abandoned by people close to you. These fears wreak havoc with relationships as you test people

**COMBINATION OF BORDERLINE PERSONALITY DISORDER AND BIPOLAR DISORDER**

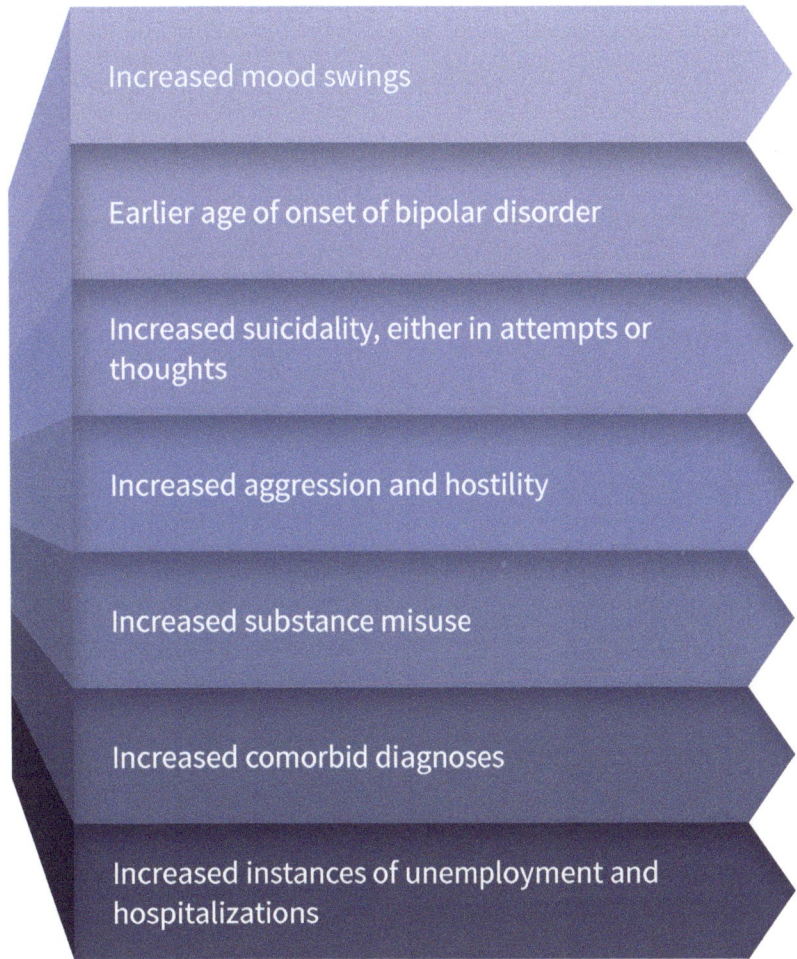

- Increased mood swings
- Earlier age of onset of bipolar disorder
- Increased suicidality, either in attempts or thoughts
- Increased aggression and hostility
- Increased substance misuse
- Increased comorbid diagnoses
- Increased instances of unemployment and hospitalizations

or sabotage the relationship to keep them from leaving you. You can engage in these behaviors even when you're not depressed or manic.

Next, the impulsivity and poor judgment you show when you're hypomanic may cause you to make bad decisions that are even worse than ones you would make if you had pure mania without the personality issues.

The feelings of emptiness intensify if you crash into a depression. This intense emptiness is one reason why there tends to be more suicidality with borderpolar than with either borderline personality disorder or bipolar alone.

Using self-harm as a coping mechanism is not a feature of bipolar disorder, but this can get out of control in a borderpolar person who's depressed or manic.

It can be complicated to recognize the interplay between both problems. When assessing these issues, a clinician will likely focus on how you have behaved in relationships over time. This is known, in psychiatry, as securing a longitudinal history. The behavior that occurs within a depression or manic episode tends to give more of a slice-in-time perspective. But behaviors that stem from your personality are present for most of your life, even when you are not depressed or manic.

If you have both disorders, you probably need a combination of medication and DBT or some other comparable therapy for your borderline personality disorder. Medication alone probably won't resolve the problem. Omitting therapy may be why we see more people with borderpolar having poor treatment outcomes. You're not likely to see much improvement if you try to address the unstable view of self and all the relationship instability with medication alone. The resulting instability leads to more depressed or angry emotions, emptiness, hopelessness, suicidal thoughts, then poor coping mechanisms like self-harm.

> **BIPOLAR DISORDER AND BORDERLINE PERSONALITY DISORDER OCCURRING TOGETHER MAKES BOTH CONDITIONS HARDER TO TREAT. COMBINATION THERAPY BECOMES VERY IMPORTANT.**

In summary, there's considerable overlap between how borderline personality disorder and bipolar disorder manifest. Sometimes, people with borderline personality disorder need the same medication that someone with bipolar disorder needs. However, bipolar disorder tends to be more episodic. In contrast, borderline personality disorder is a relatively consistent set of behaviors that can go up and down in intensity while always being present. Both disorders, though, can be treated.

## CHAPTER 23

# Bipolar Disorder vs. ADHD

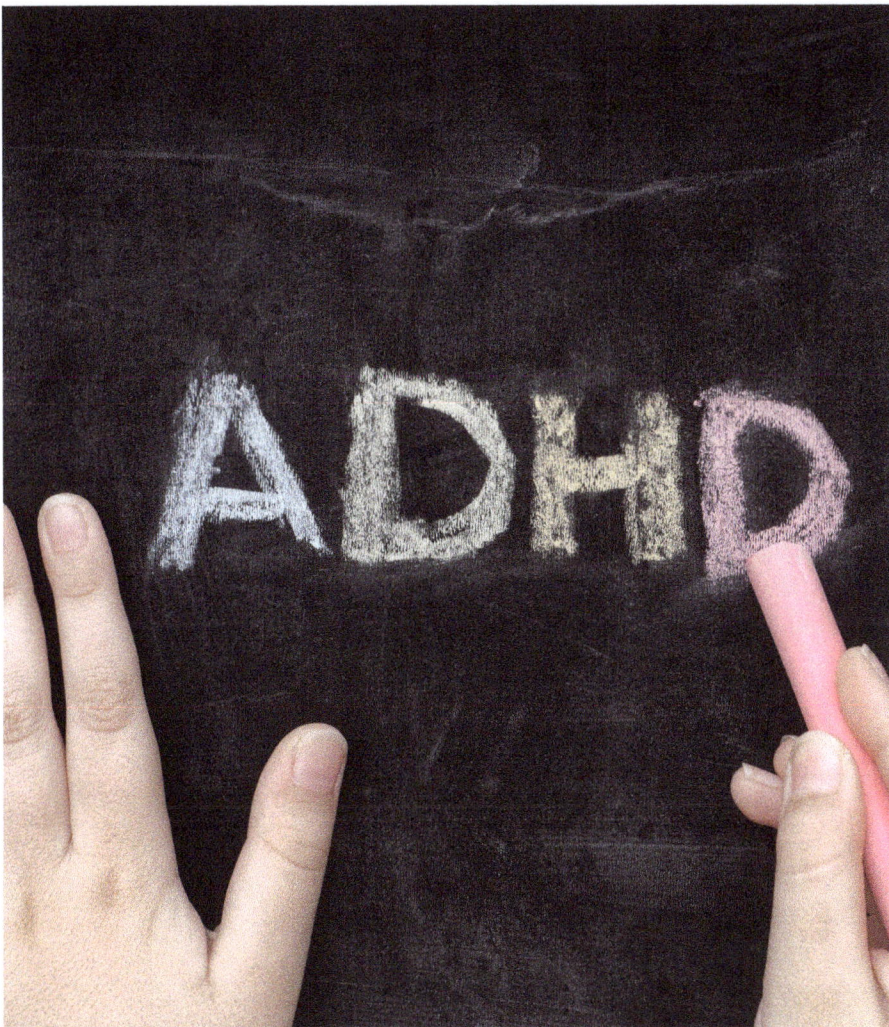

With both ADHD and bipolar disorder, you can have trouble processing thoughts, focusing, and concentrating. You can be hyperactive and yet feel disorganized. That's how these symptoms overlap. Here are some ways they differ.

Here, the terms "mania" and "hypomania" will be used interchangeably, and all of the references to mania can equally be applied to hypomania.

## ENERGY

With mania, you can feel as though you have unlimited energy. It's not just in your head. You have the ability to keep going until the episode is over. With ADHD, you may feel excited and have lots of intentions. But your energy is not unlimited. It doesn't

Attention deficit hyperactivity disorder (ADHD) and bipolar disorder can look quite similar. But they are treated very differently, so it's important to distinguish between the two disorders.

WITH ADHD YOU CAN HAVE A BUSY MIND, BUT NOT THE UNLIMITED ENERGY OF SOMEONE WITH BIPOLAR DISORDER.

have a superhuman quality.

## SPEECH

Racing thoughts and pressured speech are two symptoms of mania or hypomania. Racing thoughts is an internal experience. Your thoughts quickly move from one thing to another. Pressured speech is observable by people with whom you're communicating. The person with whom you're speaking can feel as if you're talking without any pauses, and you're difficult to interrupt. Because your thoughts are racing, you may talk over people in conversation.

ADHD is different in this respect. You interrupt people not because of fast talking and racing thoughts but because you zoned out while the person spoke and didn't realize someone else was speaking. So, you're unknowingly interrupting people in the middle of a conversation.

## MOOD

With bipolar disorder, your mood changes occur randomly and repeatedly. You can have alternating episodes

{ ADHD IS A BRAIN DISORDER THAT STARTS IN CHILDHOOD. MANY PEOPLE DON'T GET TREATMENT IN CHILDHOOD. }

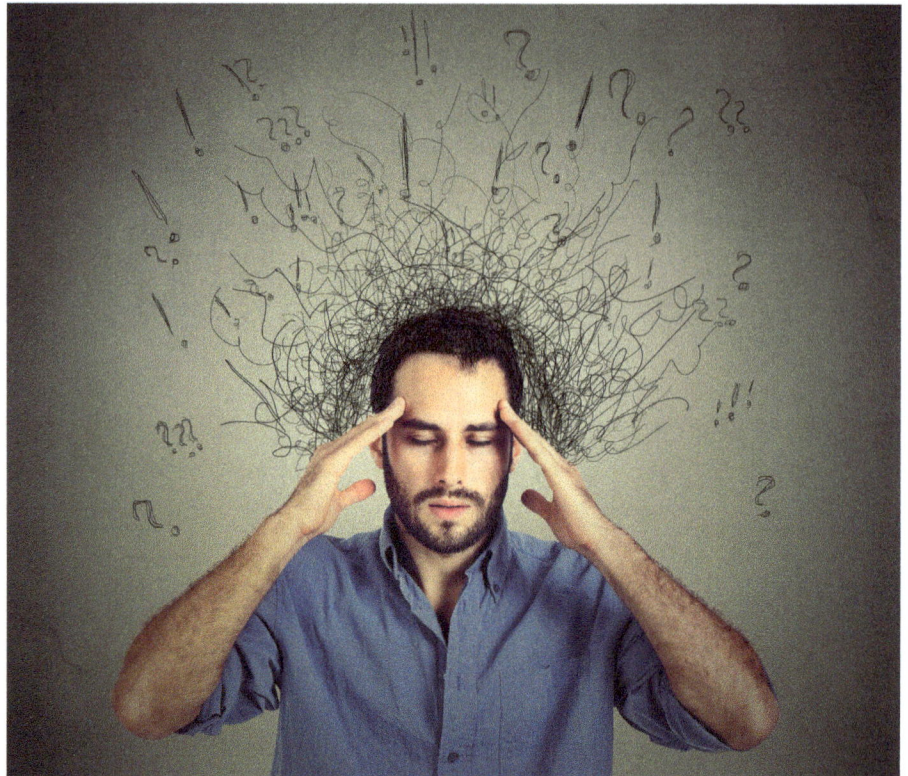

of depression and mania or recurring episodes of the same mood state.

With ADHD, any mood changes you experience are situational. Life experiences trigger them. They don't spontaneously come and go like they do with bipolar disorder.

## IMPULSIVITY

With bipolar disorder, you engage in hypersexuality and reckless spending behaviors. Someone can spend $5,000 in two days and then have no money left with which to buy groceries. A person with ADHD may make unwise decisions because they didn't think through all of the consequences. With mania, your impulsiveness continues until you have spent all your money and got into debt. You have no insight into your behavior.

With mania, you have little, if any, need for sleep, along with increased energy. You may stay up painting your home, reorganizing closets, or starting a new business. With ADHD, you may get hyper-focused on something and stay up late because you're invested in the activity. But then you're tired the next day and don't have the superhuman energy to keep going without sleep.

## AGE OF ONSET

Bipolar disorder develops over time and usually starts in the teenage years to early adulthood. There is a late-onset bipolar disorder that can happen in your fifties or sixties. Late-onset is less common, occurring in about 25% of people with bipolar disorder. Chapter 12 discusses late-onset bipolar disorder in more detail.

However, ADHD is a brain disorder beginning in childhood. Some people don't get treatment as a child, and the problem continues into adulthood. It's not until noticeable and significant problems develop that they begin taking medication, even though the problems were present to some degree earlier in childhood. You can start out having ADHD as a child and later develop bipolar disorder in addition to ADHD. In this case, you would have two comorbid conditions.

## MEDICATION RESPONSE

Bipolar disorder requires mood stabilizers to control the ups and downs. In contrast, with ADHD, your inattention, concentration, and focus respond to stimulant medication alone. If you have ADHD then later develop bipolar disorder, your ADHD challenges will be compounded by bipolar disorder. The mania can disorganize your thoughts in a way that overrides whatever effect your ADHD had on your thoughts. The mania becomes the dominant problem. So, your ADHD may no longer respond as well to stimulants alone.

Also, the stimulants can aggravate your mania by speeding you up even more. Treating poor concentration in someone with bipolar disorder and ADHD is complicated. Your ability to focus can fluctuate depending on your mood state.

You don't need mood stabilizers to help you think. Therefore, an indication that your thought problems are related to ADHD and not bipolar disorder is having your inattention resolve from the stimulant medication alone. Bipolar disorder doesn't resolve from taking a stimulant like Adderall or Ritalin.

Making this distinction between the two illnesses is something your doctor should do. But understanding some of the differences can help you communicate with your doctor about the symptoms you are experiencing.

## CHAPTER 24

# Bipolar Disorder Versus Schizoaffective Disorder

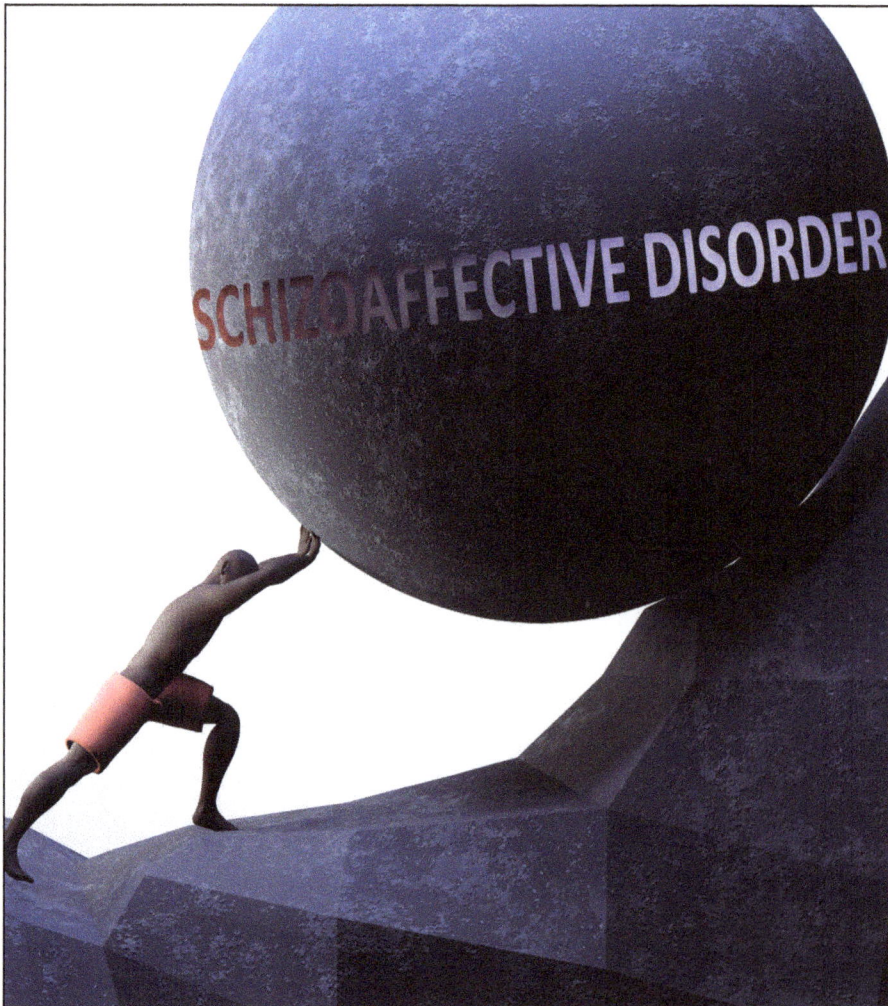

**W**here do we get the term "affective"? There's a concept called the ABCs of psychology. It divides the mind into three domains. A is for affect, which is your emotions or feelings. B is for behavior, and C is for cognition, which is how you think. Mood disorders, like depression and bipolar disorder, primarily involve changes to your emotional expression. So, they're called affective disorders.

## ABCs OF PSYCHOLOGY

**A**FFECT

**B**EHAVIOR

**C**OGNITION

By contrast, schizophrenia, at its core, affects your thinking. So it's more of a cognitive disorder. Schizoaffective disorder involves a combination of changes in your emotions and your thinking abilities.

Schizoaffective disorder is a combination of either schizophrenia and bipolar disorder or schizophrenia and depression.

Whether schizoaffective disorder should remain a separate disorder from schizophrenia is debatable. The symptoms of schizoaffective disorder look more like schizophrenia than bipolar disorder or depression. People with schizoaffective disorder are more on the schizophrenia spectrum than the mood spectrum.

Schizophrenia is a disorder where a person has psychotic symptoms as well as cognitive symptoms. The psychotic symptoms are hallucinations, delusions, and severe thought or behavioral disorganization.

A person with schizophrenia isn't necessarily depressed. They may get agitated, but this agitation is not the same as mania. Mania is an elevated or irritable mood, and many other things like increased energy and a decreased need for sleep. Someone with pure schizophrenia doesn't experience these things.

Schizoaffective disorder involves having a depressive illness or bipolar illness superimposed on schizophrenia. The clinical term is schizoaffective disorder bipolar type or depressive type.

Here's how this is different from bipolar disorder. Bipolar disorder involves having separate episodes of mania and depression. There are few, if any, symptoms when someone is in between episodes. If you did have residual symptoms, they would be associated with your last episode.

You can become psychotically depressed, or you can have mania with psychotic symptoms. In this case, though, the psychosis is a measure of the intensity of the illness, and the psychosis resolves as the episode improves.

Let's say, for instance, that you become manic and start believing you're part of a sting operation spearheaded by the CIA. The CIA has recruited you to do an investigation. During the manic episode, you stay up all night researching as part of the investigation. If you start taking medication, you may no longer believe you're part of the sting operation. But you still may have some manic symptoms like insomnia. Or you may have pressured speech and can't stop talking, but you're still thinking rationally. As your manic episode continues to resolve, everything slows back down.

Let's take the same scenario and apply it to someone with schizoaffective disorder. In this case, before becoming manic, you already believe that the CIA is gathering intelligence on people. As a result, you refuse to answer your phone because you feel that the phone is transmitting signals.

Notice that this delusion is more bizarre and unbelievable than the manic delusion.

As you lose sleep, you start believing you're being recruited to help with the surveillance. After your mania resolves, you still believe the CIA is doing something evil. Or, even if you

no longer believe the CIA story, you've moved on to a different kind of conspiracy. You continue to have this delusion for several weeks until it tapers off and you stop thinking about it. During the weeks when your conviction about the belief is diminishing, you're not depressed. Nor are you manic.

Sorting out these symptoms can get complicated because you can have schizophrenia with major depression as a second illness. The difference here is that with schizophrenia plus major depression, you spend more time with psychotic symptoms than you spend in a depression. So, you're mostly psychotic with intermittently surfacing outbreaks of depression. With schizoaffective disorder depressed type, you're both psychotic and depressed during most of the illness. But you will have psychotic symptoms before or after your mood symptoms resolve.

There are minor differences in the kind of treatment you will receive. A person with bipolar disorder is going to be on mood stabilizers.

{ SCHIZOAFFECTIVE DISORDER AFFECTS YOUR THINKING MUCH MORE SEVERELY THAN BIPOLAR DISORDER. }

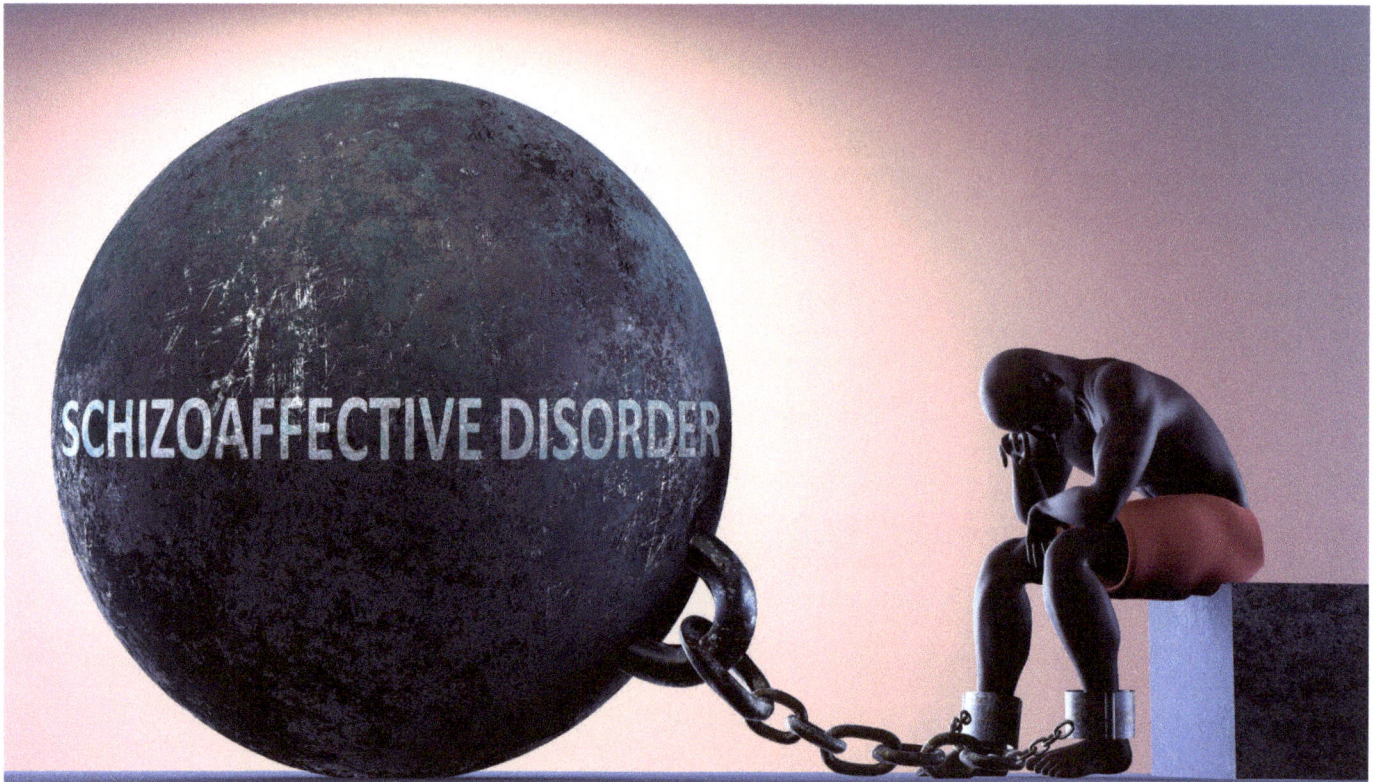

As previously discussed, medications used to treat bipolar disorder are mood stabilizers and antipsychotics. A person with bipolar disorder can be on a mood stabilizer like lamotrigine, which is not an antipsychotic. But a person with schizoaffective disorder will need to start with an antipsychotic medication because of the predominance of psychotic symptoms.

Your doctor may also add a mood stabilizer, like valproic acid or lamotrigine, to the antipsychotic to control the mood symptoms if the antipsychotic medication hasn't completely addressed the mood instability. So, there is some overlap between these illnesses and the medications you take.

The best way to think about comparing treatment for bipolar disorder and treatment for schizoaffective disorder bipolar type is that with bipolar disorder, you may or may not take antipsychotic medication. But with schizoaffective disorder, you always need to take antipsychotic medication.

THE KEY DIFFERENCE BETWEEN SCHIZOAFFECTIVE DISORDER AND BIPOLAR DISORDER IS THE PRESENCE OF PSYCHOSIS IN BETWEEN EPISODES.

## CHAPTER 25

# Mania vs. Anxiety

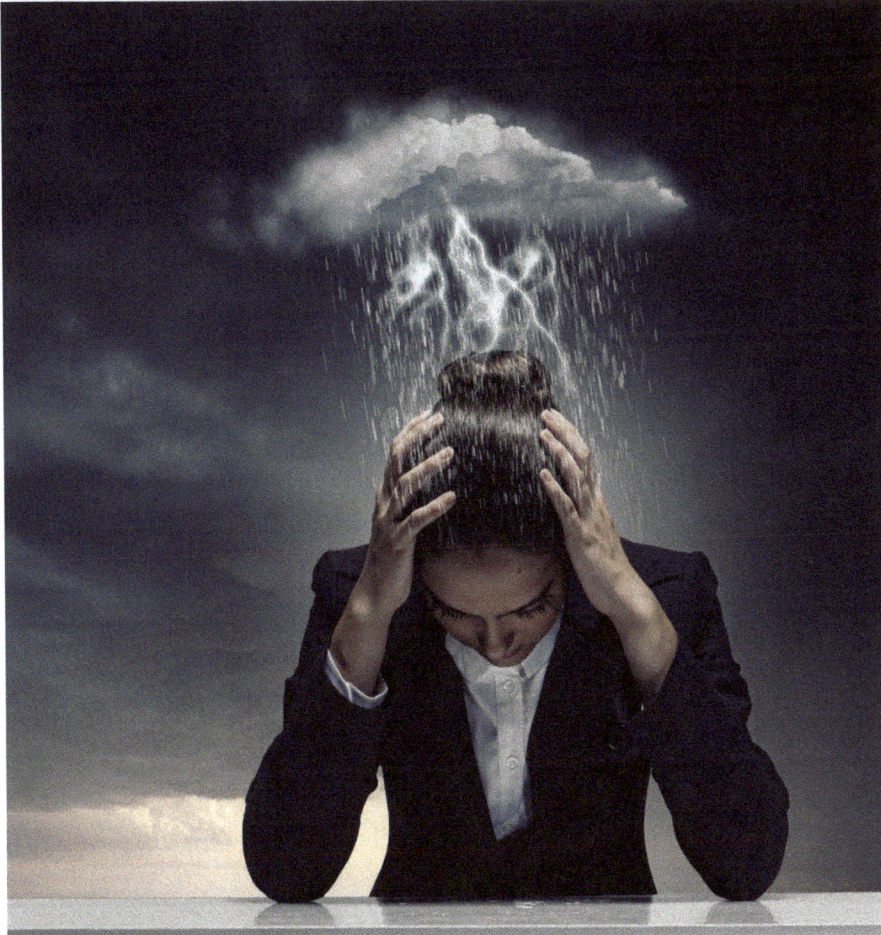

In general, anxiety is a feeling of uneasiness, fear, or dread. It can have physical manifestations, but it starts with a feeling. Mania is a state of hyperarousal. Imagine having an internal motor, and someone has turned up the dial on it. There may be emotions attached to this hyper state, but it starts with a physical acceleration.

So, in some ways, anxiety and mania can be thought of as having opposite effects. Even though anxiety and mania share some characteristics, the feelings descend upon you and affect you physically with anxiety. With mania, your physical state intensifies your feelings.

Here are the symptoms that look similar in anxiety and mania:

- Racing thoughts
- Concentration problems
- Irritability
- Inability to sleep
- Restlessness or agitation.

Here, we'll focus on generalized anxiety, where the primary manifestation is being consumed by worry and fear. Generalized anxiety disorder is one of many anxiety disorders, such as panic disorder and social phobia.

Anxiety disorders can occur along with bipolar disorder, and there is some overlap in the way anxiety and mania look. Here's why this matters. If a manic episode is coming, the intervention your doctor is most likely to make is adjusting your mood stabilizer. But you don't need to change your primary medication regimen if what you are experiencing is anxiety and not mania.

**Concentration problems**

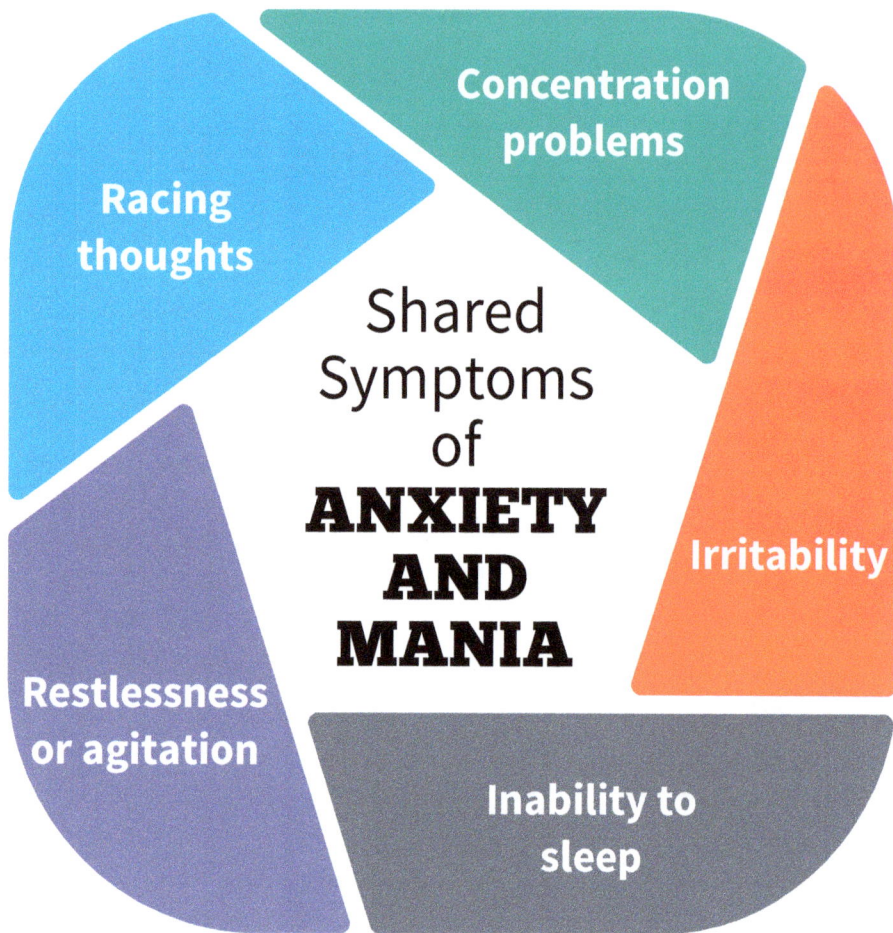

**Racing thoughts**

Shared Symptoms of **ANXIETY AND MANIA**

**Irritability**

**Restlessness or agitation**

**Inability to sleep**

after another. Also, because of the increased energy, the manic person may be speaking louder.

By contrast, the anxious person is usually suffering silently. Even if they verbalize their worries, they aren't talking loud and fast about what they're thinking.

## CONCENTRATION PROBLEMS

Here, worry and fretting interfere with your focus. You can't filter the thoughts to give your full attention to something else. You can have a similar problem with mania because your thoughts are blooming fast. Still, the main difference here is that this focus and concentration problem exists during the manic episode. When your episode resolves, you stop thinking and talking fast, and you're back to your baseline level of concentration.

Anxiety is a long-lasting, chronic condition. It comes and goes in waves throughout your life. You may have seasons where it becomes unmanageable, and then quiet periods where it's not so bad. Since you don't become entirely anxiety-free, your concentration problems can persist to a milder degree when you're not as anxious. So, anxiety involves having your concentration problems worsening or improving depending on your anxiety level.

## IRRITABILITY

Anxiety is a state of distress. It's particularly unpleasant because your brain remains in a state of

## RACING THOUGHTS

With anxiety, you have trouble shutting off your worries: you overfocus on a perceived threat. You worry, fret, and experience intrusive thoughts, which you can't get out of your mind. It can feel as though you have a recording of yourself talking about these what-if scenarios, and you can't turn off the recording. It can even keep you from falling asleep and distract you from paying attention to things in the moment.

Yet mania is different. Here, the dial on your motor has been turned up and you have increased energy, making everything move faster. You *are* producing more

thoughts, and you can't keep up. It's like being in a race where the finish line is continually moving and you can never get to the end. Imagine a time-lapse video of a blooming flower where the petals just keep coming. That's how your thoughts can feel. And the theme of what you're thinking doesn't necessarily consist of fear or worry. You can have ordinary thoughts that are just processing faster.

Just as your thoughts are moving fast, the speed of your speech matches your thoughts. You can speak in a firehose of words. We call this pressured speech. It's hard for someone else to find a natural break in your speech because it consists of one thought threat-awareness. This can make you irritable and edgy. Severe anxiety can also progress to depression.

Mania creates a certain level of disinhibition. You're not able to control your emotional reactivity. Just as your motor dial is increased, so is your sensitivity dial. So, you have more raw, unfiltered emotional reactions. It doesn't take much to transform your good (or even elated) mood into a grumpy or angry one.

## INABILITY TO SLEEP

Anxiety can disrupt your sleep by making you worry.  The anxiety keeps you awake as your mind races from one concern or fear to another. Not every anxious person sleeps poorly, but your sleep can indicate the severity of your anxiety. If you don't sleep well because of anxiety, you feel run down, especially when it happens multiple nights in a row.

Mania is associated with not needing much sleep. You may only sleep 2 hours because you were up reorganizing your shelves. But you can still feel energized by those couple of hours and can do that for several nights in a row with little difficulty.

## RESTLESSNESS OR AGITATION

Agitation is a physical state of excessive movement. An anxious person can have physical symptoms of anxiety, like feeling tense or breathing faster. You may feel like you can't relax, and you feel the need to pace to deal with your tension.

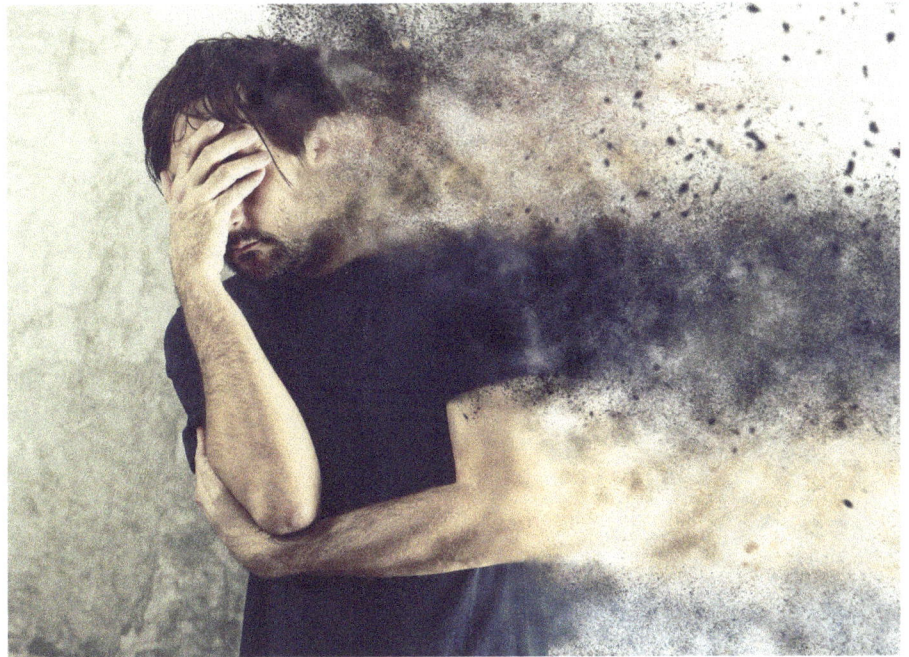

On the other hand, a manic person has energy pushing them to keep moving. If you watch a manic person, they're less likely to look like they're pacing out of worry and angst. Instead, they may look very busy sort of like a worker ant.

An exception to this is the person with mixed mania and depression, who may be tired from the depression but wired and amped up from the mania. They usually look irritable and miserable. The person with pure anxiety may be stressed and worried but not sad and miserable unless they've slid into an anxious, depressed state.

There are nuances here, but you can get a sense of the general way an anxious person looks compared to a manic person. Also, you can have bipolar disorder and anxiety, and the anxiety worsens either the depression or the mania. It can be tricky to treat an anxiety disorder when someone has a bipolar disorder because antidepressants used for anxiety can worsen bipolar disorder.

So, your doctor must carefully consider these complex factors to devise a plan of action.  Your medication plan has to take into account your current symptoms and your past response to medication. It may be the case that therapy for anxiety is the best approach to managing symptoms, reserving medication to treat the bipolar disorder.

# Conclusion

**W**e've looked at bipolar disorder, unpacked its nuances, identified proven effective treatments, and discussed how this mental health challenge intersects with others. There's no one-size-fits-all treatment regimen for this condition, and it's more common than people realize.

Doubtless, living with bipolar disorder is challenging. Thankfully, with the assistance of appropriate medical attention and a disciplined approach to finding workable solutions, you can manage this condition. Hopefully, this guide will be useful to you and will contribute to an increased awareness of the importance of understanding mental health challenges in general.

Lastly, we shouldn't let mental health challenges define who we are. Instead, we should understand them better and use that understanding to create a life that has meaning and value individually and collectively. That's what psychiatry, as a discipline and profession, seeks to accomplish, and that's what this guide is intended to achieve.

# Bibliography

## CHAPTER 1

American Psychiatric Association (2013) *Diagnostic and Statistical Manual of Mental Disorders* (5th ed.). https://doi.org/10.1176/appi.books.9780890425596

## CHAPTER 2

McGlinchey JB, Zimmerman M, Young D, et al. (2006) "Diagnosing major depressive disorder VIII: are some symptoms better than others?" *J. Nerv. Ment. Dis.*, 194(10): 785–790. doi:10.1097/01.nmd.0000240222.75201.aa

Liu RT, Kleiman EM, Nestor BA, et al. (2015) "The hopelessness theory of depression: A quarter century in review." *Clin. Psychol. (New York)*, 22(4): 345–365. doi:10.1111/cpsp.12125

Goes FS, Sadler B, Toolan J, et al. (2007) "Psychotic features in bipolar and unipolar depression." *Bipolar Disord.*, 9(8): 901–906. doi:10.1111/j.1399-5618.2007.00460.x

American Psychiatric Association (2013) *Diagnostic and Statistical Manual of Mental Disorders* (5th ed.). https://doi.org/10.1176/appi.books.9780890425596

## CHAPTER 3

Aiken CB, Weisler RH, Sachs GH (2015) "The Bipolarity index: a clinician-rated measure of diagnostic confidence." *J. Affect. Dis.*, 177: 59–64.

Lam DH, Jones SH, Hayward P (2010) *Cognitive Therapy for Bipolar Disorder: A therapist's guide to concepts, methods, and practice* (2nd ed.). John Wiley & Sons. https://doi.org/10.1002/9780470970256

## CHAPTER 5

Ghaemi SN (2013) "Bipolar spectrum: A review of the concept and a vision for the future." *Psychiatry Investig.*, 10(3): 218–224. doi:10.4306/pi.2013.10.3.218

Mondimore FM (2005) "Kraepelin and manic-depressive insanity: A historical perspective." *Int. Rev. Psychiatry*, 17(1): 49–52. doi:10.1080/09540260500080534

Trade K, Salvatore P, Baethge C, et al. (2005) "Manic-depressive illness: Evolution in Kraepelin's textbook, 1883–1926." *Harv. Rev. Psychiatry*, 13(3): 155–178. doi:10.1080/10673220500174833

Singh T, Williams K (2006) "Atypical depression." *Psychiatry (Edgmont)*, 3(4): 33–39.

## CHAPTER 6

Perugi G, Hantouche E, Vannucchi G (2017) "Diagnosis and treatment of cyclothymia: The 'primacy' of temperament." *Curr. Neuropharmacol.*, 15(3): 372–379.

Benazzi F (2009) "Cyclothymic temperament: The impact of age." *Psychopathology*, 42: 165–169. doi:10.1159/000207458

## CHAPTER 9

Fava G, Kellner R (1991) "Prodromal symptoms in affective disorders." *Am. J. Psychiatry*, 148(7): 823–830.

McAulay C, Mond J, Touyz S (2018) "Early intervention for bipolar disorder in adolescents: A psychosocial perspective." *Early Interv. Psychiatry*, 12(3): 286–291. doi:10.1111/eip.12474

## CHAPTER 13

Stanley B, Brown, G. (2011) "Safety planning intervention: A brief intervention to mitigate suicide risk." *Cogn. Behav. Pract.*, 19(2), 256–264.

## CHAPTER 14

Perugi G, Hantouche E, Vannucchi G (2017) "Diagnosis and treatment of cyclothymia: The 'primacy' of temperament." *Curr. Neuropharmacol.*, 15(3): 372–379. doi:10.2174/1570159X14666160616120157

Marneros A, Goodwin F (2005) *Bipolar Disorders: Mixed States, Rapid Cycling and Atypical Forms*. Cambridge University Press.

## CHAPTER 15

Sugawara N, Yasui-Furukori N, Ishii N, et al. (2013) "Lithium in tap water and suicide mortality in Japan." *Int. J. Environ. Res. Public Health*, 10: 6044–6048.

Kapusta ND, König D (2015) "Naturally occurring low-dose lithium in drinking water." *J. Clin. Psychiatry*, 76(3): e373–374. doi:10.4088/JCP.14com09574

Malhi GS, Tanious M, Das P. et al. (2013) "Potential mechanisms of action of lithium in bipolar disorder." *CNS Drugs*, 27(2): 135–153.

Shine B, McKnight RF, Leaver L, et al. (2015) "Long-term effects of lithium on renal, thyroid, and parathyroid function: A retrospective analysis of laboratory data." *Lancet*, 386(9992): 461–468. doi:10.1016/S0140-6736(14)61842-0

## CHAPTER 16

El-Mallakh RH, Vöhringer PA, Ostacher MM, et al. (2015) "Antidepressants worsen rapid-cycling course in bipolar depression: A STEP-BD randomized clinical trial." *J. Affect. Disord.*, 184: 318–321.

## CHAPTER 17

Douma LG, Gumz ML (2018) "Circadian clock-mediated regulation of blood pressure." *Free Radic. Biol. Med.*, 119: 108–114. doi:10.1016/j.freeradbiomed.2017.11.024

Dayabandara M, Hanwella R, Ratnatunga S, et al. (2017) "Antipsychotic-associated weight gain: Management strategies and impact on treatment adherence." *Neuropsychiatr. Dis. Treat.*, 13: 2231–2241. doi:10.2147/NDT.S113099

Mitchell AJ, Vancampfort D, De Herdt A, et al. (2013) "Is the prevalence of metabolic syndrome and metabolic abnormalities increased in early schizophrenia? A comparative meta-analysis of first episode, untreated and treated patients." *Schizophr. Bull.*, 39(2): 295–305.

Bazo-Alvarez JC, Morris TP, Carpenter JR, et al. (2020) "Effects of long-term antipsychotics treatment on body weight: A population-based cohort study." *J. Psychopharmacol.* 34(1): 79–85. doi:10.1177/0269881119885918

Feingold KR (2021) "Introduction to lipids and lipoproteins." In: Feingold KR, Anawalt B, Boyce A et al. (eds.) *Endotext* [Internet]. MDText.com, Inc.; 2000–. https://www.ncbi.nlm.nih.gov/books/NBK305896/

BMI calculator: https://www.nhlbi.nih.gov/health/educational/lose_wt/BMI/bmicalc.htm

Ban TA (2007) "Fifty years chlorpromazine: A historical perspective." *Neuropsychiatr. Dis. Treat.*, 3(4): 495–500.

Grajales D, Ferreira V, Valverde ÁM (2019) "Second-generation antipsychotics and dysregulation of glucose metabolism: Beyond weight gain." *Cells*, 8(11): 1336. doi:10.3390/cells8111336

## CHAPTER 18

Geddes JR, Miklowitz DJ (2013) "Treatment of bipolar disorder." *Lancet*, 381(9878): P1672–1682. doi:10.1016/S0140-6736(13)60857-0

Naik SK (2015) "Management of bipolar disorders in women by nonpharmacological methods." *Indian J. Psychiatry*, 57 (Suppl. 2): S264–S274. doi:10.4103/0019-5545.161490

Haynes PL, Gengler D, Kelly M (2016) "Social rhythm therapies for mood disorders: An update." *Curr. Psychiatry Rep.*, 18: 75. doi:10.1007/s11920-016-0712-3

Miklowitz DJ, Otto MW, Frank E, et al. (2007) "Psychosocial treatments for bipolar depression: A 1-year randomized trial from the Systematic Treatment Enhancement Program." *Arch. Gen. Psychiatry*, 64(4): 419–426. doi:10.1001/archpsyc.64.4.419

Frank E, Soreca I, Swartz HA, et al. (2008) "The role of interpersonal and social rhythm therapy in improving occupational functioning in patients with bipolar 1 disorder." *Am. J. Psychiatry*, 165(12): 1559–1565. doi:10.1176/appi.ajp.2008.07121953

## CHAPTER 19

Barbini B, Benedetti F, Colombo C, et al. (2005) "Dark therapy for

mania: A pilot study." *Bipolar Disord.* 7(1): 98–101. doi:10.1111/j.1399-5618.2004.00166.x

Henriksen TE, Skrede S, Fasmer OB, et al. (2016) "Blue-blocking glasses as additive treatment for mania: A randomized placebo-controlled trial." *Bipolar Disorders*, 18(3): 221–232.

Harvey AG (2008) "Sleep and circadian rhythms in bipolar disorder: Seeking synchrony, harmony, and regulation." *Am. J. Psychiatry*, 165(7): 820–829. doi:10.1176/appi.ajp.2008.08010098

Van Tienoven TP, Minnen J, Daniels S, et al. (2014) "Calculating the Social Rhythm Metric (SRM) and examining its use in Interpersonal Social Rhythm Therapy (IPSRT) in a healthy population study." *Behav. Sci. (Basel)*, 4(3): 265–277. doi:10.3390/bs4030265

Melyan Z, Tarttelin EE, Bellingham J, et al. (2005) "Addition of human melanopsin renders mammalian cells photoresponsive." *Nature*, 433: 741–745. doi:10.1038/nature03344

Shechter A, Kim EW, St-Onge MP, et al. (2018) "Blocking nocturnal blue light for insomnia: A randomized controlled trial." *J. Psychiatr. Res.*, 96: 196–202.

Antúnez JM (2020) "Circadian typology is related to emotion regulation, metacognitive beliefs, and assertiveness in healthy adults." *PLOS ONE*, 15(3): e0230169.

## CHAPTER 20

Sit DK, McGowan J, Wiltrout C, et al. (2018) "Adjunctive bright light therapy for bipolar depression: A randomized double-blind placebo-controlled trial." *Am. J. Psychiatry*, 175(2): 131–139. doi:10.1176/appi.ajp.2017.16101200

Al-Karawi D, Jubair L (2016) "Bright light therapy for nonseasonal depression: Meta-analysis of clinical trials." *J. Affect. Dis.*, 198: 64–71. doi:10.1016/j.jad.2016.03.016

Golden RN, Gaynes BN, Ekstrom RD, et al. (2005) "The efficacy of light therapy in the treatment of mood disorders: A review and meta-analysis of the evidence." *Am. J. Psychiatry*, 162(4): 656–662.

Geoffroy PA, Bellivier F, Scott J, et al. (2014) "Seasonality and bipolar disorder: A systematic review, from admission rates to seasonality of symptoms." *J. Affect. Dis.*, 168: 210–223.

Phelps J (2016) "Light box therapy: A treatment for all seasons?" *Psychiatric Times*, Dec 6. http://www.psychiatrictimes.com/bipolar-disorder/light-box-therapytreatment-all-seasons

Phelps J (2016) "New zero-risk treatment for mania." *Psychiatric Times*, Aug. 10. http://www.psychiatrictimes.com/bipolar-disorder/new-zero-risk-treatment-mania

Tseng PT, Chen YW, Tu KY, et al. (2016) "Light therapy in the treatment of patients with bipolar depression: A meta-analytic study." *Eur. Neuropsychopharmacol.*, 26(6): 1037–1047. doi:10.1016/j.euroneuro.2016.03.001

Crowley SJ, Molina TA, Burgess HJ (2015) "A week in the life of full-time office workers: Workday and weekend light exposure in summer and winter." *Appl. Ergon.*, 46 Pt. A: 193–200. doi:10.1016/j.apergo.2014.08.006

## CHAPTER 21

Bauer M, Glenn T, Alda M, et al. (2017) "Solar insolation in springtime influences age of onset of bipolar 1 disorder." *Acta Psychiatr. Scand.*, 136(6): 571–582.

## CHAPTER 22

Patel RS, Manikkara G, Chopra A (2019) "Bipolar disorder and comorbid borderline personality disorder: Patient characteristics and outcomes in US hospitals." *Medicine (Kaunas)*, 55(1): 13. doi:10.3390/medicina55010013

American Psychiatric Association (2013) *Diagnostic and Statistical Manual of Mental Disorders* (5th ed.). https://doi.org/10.1176/appi.books.9780890425596

## CHAPTER 24

Seldin K, Armstrong K, Schiff ML, et al. (2017) "Reducing the diagnostic heterogeneity of schizoaffective disorder." *Front Psychiatry*, 8: 18. doi:10.3389/fpsyt.2017.00018

Amann BL, Canales-Rodríguez EJ, Madre M, et al. (2015) "Brain structural changes in schizoaffective disorder compared to schizophrenia and bipolar disorder." *Acta Psychiatr Scand.* 133(1): 23–33. doi:10.1111/acps.12440

Hartman LI, Heinrichs RW, Mashhadi F (2019) "The continuing story of schizophrenia and schizoaffective disorder: One condition or two?" *Schizophr. Res. Cogn.* 16: 36–42. doi:10.1016/j.scog.2019.01.001

## CHAPTER 25

Perugi G, Akiskal HS, Toni C, et al. (2001) "The temporal relationship between anxiety disorders and (hypo)mania: A retrospective examination of 63 panic, social phobic and obsessive-compulsive patients with comorbid bipolar disorder." *J. Affect. Disord.* 67(1–3): 199–206. doi:10.1016/s0165-0327(01)00433-5

Keller MB (2002) "The long-term clinical course of generalized anxiety disorder." *J. Clin. Psychiatry*, 63 (Suppl. 8): 11–16.

www.ingramcontent.com/pod-product-compliance
Lightning Source LLC
Chambersburg PA
CBHW042354030426
42336CB00029B/3472